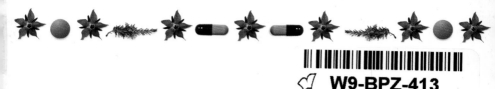

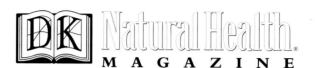

DK Natural Health® MAGAZINE

INSTANT GUIDE TO
DRUG-HERB
INTERACTIONS

By CHRIS D. MELETIS, N.D.
and the editors of *Natural Health*® Magazine
with SHEILA BUFF
Produced by The Philip Lief Group

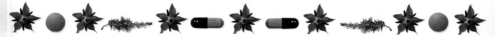

LONDON, NEW YORK, SYDNEY, DELHI, PARIS,
MUNICH, and JOHANNESBURG

Category Publisher: LaVonne Carlson
Art Director: Tina Vaughan • **Senior Editor:** Jill Hamilton
Art Editor: Megan Clayton • **Designer:** Barbara Scott-Goodman
Cover Design: Dirk Kaufman • **Production Director:** David Proffit

Natural Health® magazine is the leading publication in the field of natural self-care.
For subscription information call 800-526-8440 or visit www.naturalhealthmag.com.
Natural Health® is a registered trademark of Weider Publications, Inc.

AUTHOR'S NOTE
The author strongly recommends that you consult a conventional medical practitioner before
following any complementary therapies if you have any symptoms of illness, any diagnosed ailment,
or are receiving conventional treatment or medication for any condition. Do not cease conventional
treatment or medication without first consulting your doctor. Always inform your doctor and your
complementary practitioner of any treatments, medication, or remedies that you are taking or intend to take.

ACKNOWLEDGMENTS & PICTURE CREDITS
Dorling Kindersley would like to thank Wayne Ulrich of Wayne's Pharmacy,
Garden City, for providing the drugs shown on pages 6–9.
Main photography by Dave King. Additional photography by Steve Gorton,
Neil Fletcher and Matthew Ward. Line art illustrations by Gilly Newman.

First American Edition, 2001   10 9 8 7 6 5 4 3 2 1
Published in the United States by Dorling Kindersley Publishing, Inc.
95 Madison Avenue, New York, New York 10016

Dorling Kindersley Publishing offers special discounts for bulk purchases for sales promotions or premiums. Specific, large-
quantity needs can be met with special editions, including personalized covers, excerpts of existing guides, and corporate
imprints. For more information, contact Special Markets Department, Dorling Kindersley Publishing, Inc.,
95 Madison Avenue, New York, NY 10016 Fax: 800-600-9098.

Library of Congress cataloging-in-publication data
Natural health instant guide to drug-herb interactions
    p. cm.
  ISBN 0-7894-7150-7 (alk. paper)
    1. Drug-herb interactions.

RM302 .N38 2001
615'.7045--dc21   00-064406

Produced by The Philip Lief Group, Inc.
Reproduced by Colourscan in Singapore. Printed and bound by Artes Graficas in Spain
D.L. TO: 235-2001
See our complete catalog at **www.dk.com**

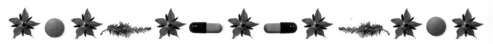

TABLE OF CONTENTS

❖

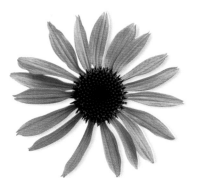

FOREWORD

ONE OF OUR MOST well-received articles at *Natural Health*® reported on dangerous interactions between drugs and herbal supplements. It was met with such an open response because using herbs to treat medical problems has become more popular than ever. In fact, according to industry statistics about one-third of all adult Americans regularly use herbs to treat health problems or maintain their health – and they spend nearly $4 billion a year on herbal products. And that's because herbs can relieve many health problems gently, safely, and effectively, without the unpleasant and even dangerous side effects caused by many prescription drugs. For example, a number of recent studies have found that St. John's wort works just as well as imipramine, a standard antidepressant drug, but without the drug's annoying side effects of sweating, dizziness, and dry mouth.

Unfortunately, the huge increase in the number of people using herbs hasn't been matched by a great educational effort to train physicians on the subject. Many doctors continue to prescribe drugs where herbs might work as well or even better. Others know little about the potential interactions between the drugs they prescribe and the herbs their patients may take. Here, too, St. John's wort is a good example. This widely used herb can prevent some drugs, such as the antiviral medicine indinavir, from working properly.

Every year, more than 100,000 people are hospitalized because of serious side effects or interactions from medications their doctors prescribe. Fortunately, serious problems from herbs and from herb-drug interactions are far less common, but they can occur. Because your doctor may not be aware of potential interactions, protecting your health is up to you.

At *Natural Health*®, we believe you should have all the information you need to combine herbs and drugs safely and effectively. Because no monthly magazine can cover all it wants to in depth, we created this book to give you the most up-to-the-minute knowledge in the most user-friendly format. We sincerely hope you'll use it to be your own health advocate.

Rachel Streit
Editor-in-Chief,
Natural Health®

INTRODUCTION

As a naturopathic physician I have countless patients who use both herbs and drugs to maintain their health. I try to monitor them closely to make sure that they don't experience any negative interactions between the two.

In this book, I've amassed the clinical information I have culled over the years. Most of the 150 medications in this book (organized by their generic name) are widely used for common health problems such as arthritis, infections, ulcers, high blood pressure, and high cholesterol. Others include a number of popular nonprescription drugs, such as acetaminophen, the generic name for Tylenol, and ibuprofen, also known as Advil.

Our understanding of drug-herb interactions has a long way to go, however. The interactions I discuss in these pages are only the ones we are aware of, the ones documented in the scientific literature. Unfortunately, not all possible interactions are known. If a drug you currently take is not listed in this book, it isn't safe to assume that there aren't any herbal interactions with it. Very possibly there are none, but it's also possible that a dangerous interaction simply hasn't been reported yet.

Not every drug-herb interaction is negative. For example, silymarin, the active compound in the herb milk thistle, may help protect against the liver damage that can occur as a side effect of some drugs, such as lovastatin, which is prescribed to lower cholesterol.

Also, do not mix herbs and drugs that have similar actions. For example, the drug diazepam is prescribed to treat anxiety. The herb kava kava is also recommended for anxiety. Combining the two could cause serious drowsiness and disorientation. Likewise, don't mix drugs and herbs that have opposite actions. When in doubt, don't combine an herb with a drug.

Be sure to tell your doctor about all the prescription and nonprescription drugs, herbs, vitamins, and minerals that you take. This can help you avoid negative reactions. Most important of all, never stop or start taking any medication – prescription drug or herbal remedy – without discussing it with your doctor.

There are other steps you can take to avert potential problems. Consult with your pharmacist; these professionals are often very knowledgeable on the subject of drug-herb interactions.

I hope this *Instant Guide to Drug-Herb Interactions* will help you avoid bad interactions. I also hope it helps you become a savvy herb user. Use it in good health!

Chris D. Meletis, N.D.
Dean of Clinical Affairs/Chief Medical Officer
National College of Naturopathic Medicine

Alendronate
Fosamax

Allopurinal
Zyloprim

Amiloride
Moduretic

Amitriptyline
Elavil

Amoxicillin
Amoxil

Atenolol
Tenormin

Atorvastatin
Lipitor

Azithromycin
Zithromax

Benazapril
Lotensin

Brompheniramine
Dimetapp

Buspirone
Buspar

Captopril
Capoten

Carbidopa
Sinemet

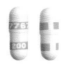

Celecoxib
Celebrex

Cephalosporins
Cephalexin

Cetrizine
Zyrtec

Ciprofloxacin
Cipro

Clarithromycin
Biaxin

Conjugated Estrogen
Premarin

Diazepam
Valium

Digoxin
Lanoxin

Erythromycin
E-mycin

Fluoxetine
Prozac

Fluvastatin
Lescol

Furosemide
Lasix

Glipizide
Glucotrol

Glyburide
Micronase

Lansoprazole
Prevacid

Levothyroxine
Synthroid

Lisinopril
Prinivil

Lovastatin
Mevacor

Loratidine
Claritin

Metformin
Glucophage

Nifedipine
Procardia

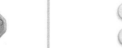

Nizatidine
Axid

Omeprazole
Prilosec

Paroxetine
Paxil

Pravastatin
Pravachol

Prednisone
Deltasore

Progesterone
Prometrium

Quinapril
Accupril

Ramipril
Altace

Ranitidine
Zantac

Sertraline
Zoloft

Simvastatin
Zocor

Venlafaxine
Effexor

Warfarin
Coumadin

Zolpidem
Ambien

Sectral

ACEBUTOLOL

Type of Drug:	Beta blocker
Description:	Acebutolol is used to treat high blood pressure and abnormal heart rhythms. It is a powerful drug that can interact adversely with a number of prescription drugs; it must be used with caution. Be certain to tell your doctor about any other prescription and nonprescription drugs and dietary supplements you are taking. The antacid cimetidine (see page 41) and related antacids, known as H2-antagonists, such as famotidine (see page 76) and ranitidine (see page 138), increase the amount of acebutolol absorbed from the gut into the bloodstream, thus increasing blood levels of this drug. Ask your doctor or pharmacist to help you choose a different type of antacid.
Don't Mix With:	No known herbal interactions. However, because acebutolol has so many potential drug interactions, avoid taking any herbal supplements, unless recommended by your physician.
Bear in Mind:	Beta blockers impede your body's use of coenzyme Q10, (also known as CoQ10 or ubiquinone) which is needed for energy production within your cells. Consider CoQ10 supplements (20-50 mg daily).

Anacin 3, Aspirin-Free Excedrin, Bayer Select, Excedrin PM, Panadol, Tylenol, others

ACETAMINOPHEN

Type of Drug:	Pain reliever and fever reducer
Description:	Acetaminophen is used to relieve fever and pain. It does not relieve inflammation. Acetaminophen is sold as a nonprescription drug, and is also used in many nonprescription drug combinations for treating pain, fever, and the symptoms of colds and flu. As a prescription drug for pain it is usually used in combination with powerful narcotics. Note that, although acetaminophen is very widely used, there is a risk of liver damage if this drug is taken in large doses for long periods of time (a year or longer).
Don't Mix With:	No known herbal interactions.
Do Take With:	Milk thistle (*Silybum marianum*). Silymarin, the active compound in milk thistle, may help prevent liver damage from long-term use of acetaminophen. Consider 150 mg, three to four times daily. Schisandra (*Schisandra chinensis*). Animal studies show that a compound in this herb may help prevent liver damage caused by long-term use of acetaminophen. Consider 250 mg, once or twice daily.
Bear in Mind:	To avoid the possibility of liver damage, do not drink alcohol while you are taking acetaminophen. According to a 1976 study, very large doses of vitamin C (over 3 grams a day) may increase the levels of acetaminophen in your bloodstream by reducing the rate at which your body excretes the drug. As a result, you could take less of the drug, but you could accidentally take too much. Both coenzyme Q10 (Co Q10 or ubiquinone) and the amino acid methionine may help prevent liver damage from long-term use of acetaminophen. Consider 20-50 mg coenzyme Q10 daily or 250 mg methionine daily.

Dazamide, Diamox

ACETAZOLAMIDE

Type of Drug:	Carbonic anhydrase inhibitor diuretic
Description:	Acetazolamide is prescribed for some people with glaucoma, because it helps reduce pressure inside the eye. It is sometimes used to treat certain forms of epilepsy, altitude sickness, as well as heart disease.

Don't Mix With:

Herbal diuretics. Avoid herbal diuretics including bilberry leaf (*Vaccinium myrtillus*), buchu (*Barosma betulina*), burdock (*Arctium lappa*), couch grass (*Agropyron repens*), damiana (*Turnera diffusa*), dandelion (*Taraxacum officinale*), fennel seed (*Foeniculum vulgare*), goldenrod (*Solidago virgaurea*), horsetail (*Equisetum arvense*), kava kava (*Piper methysticum*), kola nut (*Cola spp.*), marshmallow (*Althaea officinalis*), maté (*Ilex paraguariensis*), parsley (*Petroselinum*), sarsaparilla (*Smilax spp.*), saw palmetto (*Serenoa repens*), uva ursi (*Arctostaphylos uva ursi*), vervain (*Verbena spp.* and *V. hastata*), and yarrow (*Achillea millefolium*). Any other prescription or nonprescription diuretics should also be avoided, except on medical advice.

Herbal stimulants. Because stimulants can make glaucoma worse, avoid caffeine, ephedra (*Ephedra spp.*), ginseng (*Panax ginseng*), guaraná (*Paullinia cupana*), kola nut (*Cola spp.*), maté (*Ilex paraguariensis*), sarsaparilla (*Smilax spp.*), yohimbe (*Pausinystalia yohimbe*), and all other herbal stimulants.

Salicylate-containing herbs. The herbs white willow bark (*Salix spp.*) and meadowsweet (*Filipendula ulmaria*) interact adversely with acetazolamide. Note that aspirin is a salicylate-containing drug; discuss alternatives to aspirin and aspirin-like drugs with your doctor.

Bear in Mind:

Acetazolamide can decrease the potassium in your body. Eating two servings a day of potassium-rich foods (bananas, kiwis, oranges and other citrus fruits, and tomatoes) helps replace the lost potassium; your doctor may prescribe a potassium supplement.

Zovirax

ACYCLOVIR

Type of Drug:	Antiviral
Description:	Acyclovir is used to treat herpes simplex, shingles, chickenpox, and some other viral infections. It is usually used as an ointment applied to the skin; pills are generally prescribed only for patients who have frequent flare-ups of herpes blisters.
Don't Mix With:	No known herbal interactions.
Bear in Mind:	The amino acid arginine seems to encourage the growth of the herpes virus. Avoiding foods high in arginine, such as chocolate, wheat, oats, peanuts, nuts, and beer, may help prevent a flare-up. The amino acid lysine seems to inhibit the growth of the herpes virus. Eating foods rich in lysine, such as fish, chicken, lean meat, milk, and cheese, may help reduce the severity of a herpes flare-up. Consider lysine supplements (2,000 to 3,000 mg daily).

Proventil, Ventolin, Volmax

ALBUTEROL

Type of Drug:	Bronchodilator
Description:	Albuterol is used to treat and prevent asthma attacks. It is usually inhaled, but it can also be used in tablet form.
Don't Mix With:	Digitalis (*Digitalis spp.*, also known as foxglove, and *D. lanata*). This dangerous herb is very similar to the heart drug digoxin, which was originally derived from the plant. One study showed that albuterol reduces digoxin levels. Until more is known, don't take digitalis and albuterol concurrently.
Bear in Mind:	Several reports suggest that albuterol can lower your levels of calcium, magnesium, and potassium. The reports all involve albuterol that was given intravenously, by injection, or orally; none involved inhaled albuterol. However, whatever form you're taking, be sure you're getting enough of these minerals by eating foods rich in calcium (such as dairy products and fortified soy products), magnesium (such as nuts, beans, and dark-green leafy vegetables), and potassium (such as bananas, citrus fruits, beans, potatoes, and tomatoes).

Fosamax

ALENDRONATE

Type of Drug:	Bisphosphonate
Description:	Alendronate is used to treat and prevent osteoporosis.
Don't Mix With:	No known herbal interactions.
Bear in Mind:	Alendronate should be taken on an empty stomach. Food or drink (aside from plain water) sharply reduce the absorption of this drug. Both calcium supplements and the magnesium found in some antacids, such as Mylanta, may interfere with your absorption of alendronate. To be on the safe side, wait at least two hours after taking aldentronate before using antacids or supplements. Alendronate can cause abdominal pain and stomach ulcers. Taking aspirin or other anti-inflammatory drugs in addition to alendronate can increase the chances of developing stomach and intestinal problems. Bromelain, an enzyme derived from pineapple, and betaine HCl, a digestive supplement, can also cause digestive irritation when taken in conjunction with alendronate.

Lopurin, Zurinol Purinol, Zyloprim

ALLOPURINOL

Type of Drug:	Antigout medication
Description:	Allopurinol is used to treat gout, a very painful form of arthritis caused by too much uric acid in the blood. Taking allopurinol with ACE inhibitor drugs, such as captopril or enalapril, can cause a dangerous interaction. Be certain to tell your doctor if you take any medication for high blood pressure.
Don't Mix With:	No known herbal interactions.
Bear in Mind:	People with gout tend to have very more acidic urine. Taking large doses of vitamin C can make your urine even more acidic, which could lead to an increased risk of kidney stones, according to some studies. The role of vitamin C in causing kidney stones is controversial, however. Discuss supplements with your doctor. Taking large doses of folic acid supplements may help lower uric acid levels. Discuss folic acid supplements with your doctor before you try them.

Symmetrel

AMANTADINE

Type of Drug:	Antiparkinsonism and antiviral medication
Description:	Amantadine is prescribed for several different reasons. It is used to treat and prevent flu, particularly in elderly patients, to treat Parkinson's disease, and sometimes to treat multiple sclerosis.
Don't Mix With:	No known herbal interactions.
Bear in Mind:	Common side effects of amantadine include nausea, dizziness, and light-headedness. Alcohol worsens these side effects and should be avoided when taking amantadine.

Midamor, Moduretic

AMILORIDE

Type of Drug:	Potassium-sparing diuretic
Description:	Amiloride is used primarily to treat high blood pressure and congestive heart failure by reducing the amount of water in your body.

Don't Mix With:

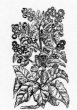

Digitalis (*Digitalis spp.*, also known as foxglove). This dangerous herb, from which the drug digoxin is derived, interacts with triamterene (see page 153) – a drug similar to amiloride – to increase the risk of body fluid imbalance. Until further information is available, do not use digitalis when taking amiloride.

Herbal diuretics. Avoid herbal diuretics including bilberry leaf (*Vaccinium myrtillus*), buchu (*Barosma betulina*), burdock (*Arctium lappa*), couch grass (*Agropyron repens*), damiana (*Turnera diffusa*), dandelion (*Taraxacum officinale*), fennel seed (*Foeniculum vulgare*), goldenrod (*Solidago virgaurea*), horsetail (*Equisetum arvense*), kava kava (*Piper methysticum*), kola nut (*Cola spp.*), marshmallow (*Althaea officinalis*), maté (*Ilex paraguariensis*), parsley (*Petroselinum spp.*), sarsaparilla (*Smilax spp.*), saw palmetto (*Serenoa repens*), uva ursi (*Arctostaphylos uva ursi*), vervain (*Verbena spp.*), and yarrow (*Achillea millefolium*). Any other prescription or nonprescription diuretics should also be avoided, except on medical advice.

Bear in Mind:

In animal studies, potassium-sparing diuretics caused an increase in magnesium levels. Although it is unknown if this can happen in humans, magnesium supplements should be avoided.

Because amiloride is a potassium-sparing diuretic, your potassium level may rise. Don't take potassium supplements, don't use salt substitutes (they are generally high in potassium), and discuss your intake of high-potassium foods, such as bananas and orange juice, with your medical practitioner.

Cordarone, Pacerone

AMIODARONE

Type of Drug:	Antiarrhythmic
Description:	Amiodarone is prescribed for life-threatening abnormal heart rhythms that haven't responded to other treatments. It is a very powerful drug that causes side effects in about 75 percent of the patients who use it. Some of the side effects can be very serious, including potentially fatal lung problems. Amiodarone can also cause dangerous interactions with a long list of drugs.
Don't Mix With:	No known herbal interactions. However, because amiodarone has so many potential drug interactions, avoid taking any herbal supplements before discussing them with your physician.
Bear in Mind:	Although the research is limited, taking vitamin E could help prevent lung damage caused by amiodarone. Discuss vitamin E supplements with your doctor before you try them.

Elavil

AMITRIPTYLINE

Type of Drug:	Tricyclic antidepressant
Description:	Amitriptyline is used to treat depression. Like other tricyclic anti-depressants, it works by affecting the way chemicals called neuro-transmitters, including serotonin and norepinephrine, move in and out of your nerve endings.

Don't Mix With:

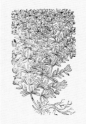

Ephedra (*Ephedra spp.*, also known as ma huang). Taking ephedra with any tricyclic antidepressant raises your risk of serious high blood pressure and heart arrhythmias. Also avoid the drugs ephedrine and pseudoephedrine, which are similar to ephedra and found in many nonprescription cold and allergy remedies.

Kava kava (*Piper methysticum*). This herbal relaxant may increase the side effects of amitriptyline.

St. John's wort (*Hypericum perforatum*). No interactions have been reported between this herb and amitriptyline, but research suggests that they work in similar ways. To avoid increasing the effects and side effects of the drug, don't take St. John's wort.

Yohimbe (*Pausinystalia yohimbe*). This dangerous herb, taken to improve male sexual function, can cause a dangerous increase in blood pressure when combined with amitriptyline.

Bear in Mind:

Heart problems can be a side effect of tricyclic antidepressants, possibly because these drugs lower the production of coenzyme Q10. Consider supplements (20 to 50 mg daily).

Although there are no studies, supplements of both s-adenylmethio-nine (SAMe) and the amino acid tryptophan (sold as 5-HTP) may increase the side effects of amitriptyline. Until more is known, do not take either concurrently with amitriptyline.

Test-tube studies indicate that tea could interfere with your absorption of amitriptyline. Don't drink tea within two hours of taking the drug.

Amoxil, Trimox, Wymox

AMOXICILLIN

Type of Drug:	Penicillin antibiotic
Description:	Amoxicillin is a form of the antibiotic penicillin. In general, penicillin antibiotics kill the bacteria that cause infections and illness. They do not kill viruses, so they are not helpful for colds and flu. Amoxicillin is often prescribed to treat ear infections in children.
Don't Mix With:	No known herbal interactions.
Bear in Mind:	Amoxicillin kills not only the harmful bacteria that cause illness but also the good bacteria that are normally found in the intestines; this can cause diarrhea. Two recent studies have shown that taking a probiotic supplement that contains Saccharomyces boulardii can help prevent or reduce the diarrhea. Consider taking probiotic supplements that contain a mix of organisms including *Saccharomyces boulardii*, *Lactobacillus acidophilus*, and *Bifido bacterium bifidum* (at least 1.5 billion live organisms daily). An enzyme found in pineapples, bromelain, increases the absorption of amoxicillin. This may be helpful for people with severe infections or infections that are not responding to amoxicillin. Discuss bromelain with your doctor before you try it.

Marcillin, Omnipen, Principen, Totacillin

AMPICILLIN

Type of Drug:	Pencillin antibiotic
Don't Mix With:	Ampicillin is similar to Amoxicillin in its description and reactions with herbs (see above for details); however, it may reduce the effect of the blood pressure-lowering drug atenolol (see page 23).

Anacin, Bayer, Bufferin, Ecotrin, Empirin, others

ASPIRIN

Type of Drug:	Pain reliever, fever reducer, and nonsteroidal anti-inflammatory drug
Description:	Aspirin, also known as acetylsalicylic acid, is one of the most commonly used nonprescription drugs in the world. Studies have shown that long-term use of low-dose aspirin can reduce your risk of heart disease and stroke and may protect against Alzheimer's disease and some forms of cancer.
	Aspirin must be used with caution. Long-term use of aspirin can cause stomach irritation, gastrointestinal bleeding, and ulcers. It can also cause bleeding problems, particularly in people who also take blood-thinning medications.
	Do not give aspirin to children and teenagers. Reye syndrome, a rare but serious childhood illness, is associated with aspirin use.
Don't Mix With:	Garlic (*Allium sativum*). Large amounts of garlic combined with aspirin may increase your risk of internal bleeding.
	Ginkgo (*Ginkgo biloba*). Taking this herb with aspirin may increase your risk of internal bleeding.
Do Take With:	Deglycyrrhizinated licorice (DGL, derived from *Glycyrrhiza glabra*). DGL can help prevent stomach irritation from aspirin. Consider taking supplements (250 mg two to three times daily).
Bear in Mind:	Taking aspirin with vitamin E or bromelain may increase the risk of internal bleeding. Mixing alcohol and aspirin can increase the risk of stomach irritation and ulcers.
	Long-term use of aspirin can lower your folic acid and vitamin C levels. Consider taking supplements (400 to 800 mcg folate and 500 mg vitamin C daily).
	High doses of aspirin (more than 3 grams a day) can reduce zinc levels. Consider taking supplements (10 mg daily, taken with food to avoid stomach upset).

Tenormin

ATENOLOL

Type of Drug:	Beta blocker
Description:	Atenolol is used primarily to treat high blood pressure, abnormal heart rhythms, and angina. It is often prescribed for people who have already had a heart attack, to help prevent another one. Atenolol interacts adversely with a number of prescription drugs. Be certain to tell your doctor about any other prescription and nonprescription drugs and dietary supplements you take. The antacid cimetidine (see page 41) and related antacids known as H2 antagonists, such as famotidine (see page 76) and ranitidine (see page 138), increase the amount of atenolol in your bloodstream. Ask your doctor or pharmacist to help you choose a different type of antacid.
Don't Mix With:	No known herbal interactions.
Bear in Mind:	Alcohol can worsen the side effects of atenolol such as drowsiness and dizziness. Beta blockers impede your body's use of coenzyme Q10, which is needed for energy production within your cells. Consider taking supplements (20-50 mg daily).

Lipitor

ATORVASTATIN

Type of Drug:	Statin cholesterol–lowering agent
Description:	Atorvastatin is prescribed to reduce high cholesterol, to slow or prevent hardening of the arteries, and to reduce the risk of heart attack and stroke.
Don't Mix With:	No known herbal interactions.
Do Take With:	Milk thistle (*Silybum marianum*). Although there are no studies to date, silymarin, the active compound in the herb milk thistle, may protect against the liver damage that can occur as a side effect of this type of drug. Consider taking supplements (150 mg three to four times daily).
Bear in Mind:	The dietary supplement, red yeast rice, sold as Cholestin, works in a way similar to the statin drugs. Do not use red yeast rice with atorvastatin. Lovastatin (see page 103), a drug similar to atorvastatin, interacts adversely with grapefruit juice. There are no studies yet of atorvastatin and grapefruit juice, but similar problems are possible. Until more is known, do not take atorvastatin with grapefruit juice. High doses of niacin (2 to 3 grams daily) can lower cholesterol levels. Combining high-dose niacin with atorvastatin, however, can lead to a serious muscle disorder. The niacin in a daily multivitamin or B vitamin supplement does not cause problems, though. According to one study, statin drugs can gradually raise vitamin A levels. Until more is known, don't take vitamin A supplements. Several studies show that taking statin drugs can significantly lower your level of coenzyme Q10 (CoQ10 or ubiquinone), a substance needed for energy production in your cells. Consider taking supplements (100 mg daily).

Donnatal, Barbidonna, others

ATROPINE

Type of Drug:	Anticholinergic combination
Description:	Atropine, in combination with other anticholinergic and sedative drugs, is used to relieve stomach and intestinal cramps. It is also used to relieve diarrhea and excessive salivation, and to treat some heart conditions.
Don't Mix With:	Tannin-containing herbs. Herbs that are high in tannin, including black walnut (*Juglans nigra*), red raspberry (*Rubus idaeus*), oak (*Quercus spp.*), uva ursi (*Arctostaphylos uva ursi*), and witch hazel (*Hamamelis virginiana*), can interfere with your absorption of atropine, as can tea.
Bear in Mind:	Do not use atropine products to treat diarrhea in babies. Adults who have diarrhea for more than three days should consult a doctor.
Also Called:	HYOSCYAMINE, SCOPALAMINE

Zithromax
AZITHROMYCIN

Type of Drug:	Macrolide antibiotic
Description:	Azithromycin is used to treat bacterial infections. It is often prescribed for middle ear infections, tonsillitis, pharyngitis, respiratory tract infections, and sexually transmitted diseases. If you take any statin drug such as lovastatin (see page 103) or atorvastatin (see page 24), do not take azithromycin. The combination could cause a potentially fatal muscle disease.
Don't Mix With:	Digitalis (*Digitalis spp.*, also known as foxglove). Antibiotics very similar to azithromycin raise your level of both the dangerous herb digitalis and digoxin, a drug with similar effects. No studies show a similar effect from azithromycin, but until more is known, don't combine the two.
Bear in Mind:	Azithromycin kills not only the harmful bacteria that cause illness but also the good bacteria that are normally found in your intestines, which can then cause diarrhea. Consider probiotic supplements (at least 1.5 billion live organisms daily, including a mixture of *Lactobacillus acidophilus, Bifidobacterium,* and *Saccharomyces boulardii*).

Retrovir

AZT (AZIDOTHYMIDINE OR ZIDOVUDINE)

Type of Drug:	Antiviral
Description:	AZT is used in combination with the protease inhibitor indinavir (see page 91) as part of a "cocktail" of pharmaceuticals to treat HIV infection and AIDS. It is very powerful and can interact badly with a number of other drugs. Be certain to tell your doctor about any other prescription and nonprescription drugs and dietary supplements you take.
Don't Mix With:	St. John's wort (*Hypericum perforatum*). The effectiveness of protease inhibitors is seriously reduced by this herb. Do not take AZT with St. John's wort.
Bear in Mind:	Naringinen, a substance found in grapefruits and grapefruit juice, may raise your blood levels of AZT too high. Don't consume grapefruits or grapefruit juice when taking AZT.
	Supplements of the amino acid carnitine may help prevent muscle pain and damage from AZT. Consider supplements (250 mg two to four times daily, or according to your doctor's recommendation). According to one study, HIV-positive people with low levels of vitamin B12 are more likely to develop anemia and other side effects from AZT. Discuss vitamin B12 supplements with your doctor before you try them (The recommended dosage is 500 mcg daily). Vitamin E may help AZT work better, according to another study. Discuss vitamin E supplements with your doctor before you try them (recommended dosage is 400 IU daily). A few studies suggest that AZT lowers your zinc and copper levels. In 1995 a study found that high doses of zinc (200 mg daily) may help prevent respiratory infections in people with AIDS. Discuss zinc supplements with your doctor before you try them. When taking large doses of zinc, additional copper (1 to 2 mg daily) is also needed.

Accupril (quinapril), Altace (ramipril), Capoten (captopril),
Lotensin (benazepril), Prinivil (lisinopril), Zestril (lisinopril),

BENAZEPRIL, CAPTOPRIL, LISINOPRIL, QUINAPRIL, RAMIPRIL

Type of Drug:	Angiotensin-converting enzyme (ACE) inhibitor
Description:	All of these drugs are part of the group known as ACE inhibitors, prescribed to treat high blood pressure, some types of heart failure, and kidney disease caused by diabetes.
Don't Mix With:	Cayenne (*Capsicum frutescens*). Capsaicin, in cayenne pepper capsules, may worsen coughing, a side effect of ACE inhibitors.
	Digitalis (*Digitalis spp.*, also known as foxglove). Similar to the heart drug digoxin (derived from the plant), which is excreted more slowly when you use ACE inhibitors, thereby raising the level of digoxin in your blood. Don't take digitalis while taking these drugs.
	Herbal diuretics. Avoid bilberry leaf (*Vaccinium myrtillus*), buchu (*Barosma betulina*), burdock (*Arctium lappa*), couch grass (*Agropyron repens*), damiana (*Turnera diffusa*), dandelion (*Taraxacum officinale*), fennel seed (*Foeniculum vulgare*), goldenrod (*Solidago virgaurea*), horsetail (*Equisetum arvense*), kava kava (*Piper methysticum*), kola nut (*Cola spp.*), marshmallow (*Althaea officinalis*), maté (*Ilex paraguariensis*), parsley (*Petroselinum spp.*), sarsaparilla (*Smilax spp.*), saw palmetto (*Serenoa repens*), uva ursi (*Arctostaphylos uva ursi*), vervain (*Verbena spp.*), and yarrow (*Achillea millefolium*), as well as other diuretics.
Bear in Mind:	ACE inhibitors may raise blood potassium levels, especially with kidney disease. Do not use potassium supplements or potassium-containing salt substitutes. Discuss high-potassium foods with your doctor.
	High doses of the amino acid arginine, with an ACE inhibitor, may affect potassium levels unpredictably. Do not take arginine supplements while taking these drugs.

Pepto-Bismol, Bismatrol, others

BISMUTH, BISMUTH SUBSALICYLATE

Type of Drug:	Antacid and antidiarrheal
Description:	Bismuth subsalicylate is a nonprescription drug used to relieve indigestion, nausea, stomach cramps, and diarrhea, especially traveler's diarrhea. It is also often used in combination with prescription drugs to treat ulcers.
Don't Mix With: 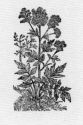	Salicylate-containing herbs. The herbs meadowsweet (*Filipendula ulmaria*), white willow bark (*Salix alba*), and wintergreen (*Gaultheria procumbens*) contain salicylates. Taking these herbs with bismuth subsalicylate could, at least in theory, make your salicylate level rise too high. This could cause blood-thinning and bleeding problems, especially if you also take blood-thinning natural substances like garlic (*Allium sativum*), ginkgo (*Ginkgo biloba*), and vitamin E, or a blood-thinning drug such as warfarin (see page 156).

Allent, Bromfed, Dimetapp Allergy, Endafed, DayQuil Allergy Relief, others

BROMPHENIRAMINE

Type of Drug:	Antihistamine
Description:	Brompheniramine is a nonprescription drug used to treat symptoms of seasonal allergies, including sneezing, runny nose, and itchy and watering eyes. It is also used to treat the symptoms of colds and upper respiratory infections, including scratchy throat and nasal congestion. In nonprescription allergy and cold formulas, brompheniramine is combined with a decongestant drug such as pseudoephedrine (see page 136). Decongestant drugs should be avoided by people with diabetes, heart disease, high blood pressure, and many other health problems. Read the label carefully.
Don't Mix With:	Henbane (*Hyoscyamus niger*). This herb is toxic and should be used only when prescribed and closely monitored by a qualified practitioner. Because brompheniramine and henbane have similar side effects, such as dry mouth, dizziness, and drowsiness, they should never be used in combination with each other.
Bear in Mind:	Brompheniramine causes drowsiness. Since alcohol can make the drowsiness worse, and because alcohol may also interact adversely with other ingredients in the formula, do not use it when taking this drug.

Wellbutrin, Zyban

BUPROPION

Type of Drug:	Antidepressant and smoking-cessation drug
Description:	As Wellbutrin, bupropion is used to treat major depression, usually when other drugs haven't helped. As Zyban, bupropion is used to help people stop smoking without gaining weight. Because bupropion can cause convulsions, it should not be used by anyone with a history of seizure disorders. This drug also often causes appetite loss, among other side effects, and can interact adversely with other drugs. Be certain to tell your doctor about any other prescription and nonprescription drugs and dietary supplements you take.
Don't Mix With:	Sedative herbs. When combined with bupropion sedative herbs may cause excessive drowsiness. Avoid sedative herbs such as chamomile (*Matricaria recutita*), catnip (*Nepeta cataria*), kava kava (*Piper methysticum*), passionflower (*Passiflora incarnata*), St. John's wort (*Hypericum perforatum*), valerian (*Valeriana officinalis*), and others, as well as sedative dietary supplements such as 5-HTP, tryptophan, and SAMe.
Bear in Mind:	Bupropion causes drowsiness and dizziness. Because alcohol can worsen these side effects, don't use it when taking this drug.

BuSpar

BUSPIRONE

Type of Drug:	Anti-anxiety
Description:	Buspirone is prescribed for treating anxiety; it is also sometimes prescribed for treating premenstrual syndrome (PMS).
Don't Mix With:	Sedative herbs. When combined with buspirone sedative herbs may cause excessive drowsiness. Avoid sedative herbs such as chamomile (*Matricaria recutita),* catnip (*Nepeta cataria*), kava kava (*Piper methysticum*), passionflower (*Passiflora incarnata*), St. John's wort (*Hypericum perforatum*), valerian (*Valeriana officinalis*), and others, as well as sedative dietary supplements such as 5-HTP, tryptophan, and SAMe.
Bear in Mind:	Buspirone is not a sedative, but it can still cause drowsiness. Because alcohol can make this side effect worse, don't use it when taking this drug.

Anacin, Caffedrine, Excedrin, Midol Max-Strength, NoDoz, Vanquish, Vivarin, others

CAFFEINE

Type of Drug:	Stimulant
Description:	Caffeine stimulates your central nervous system and helps you stay awake and alert. As a nonprescription drug (Caffedrine, NoDoz, Vivarin), caffeine is a mild stimulant. In combination with aspirin, it is a nonprescription drug for headaches and pain (Anacin, Excedrin, Midol Max-Strength, Vanquish). Caffeine is also found in a number of prescription pain drugs.
Don't Mix With:	Ephedra (*Ephedra spp.*, also known as ma huang). The stimulant herb ephedra is sold to aid weight loss and provide quick energy. It is also used for upper respiratory problems, congestion and asthma. Use ephedra with caution and do not mix it with caffeine. Guaraná (*Paullinia cupana*). The South American herb guaraná is very high in a caffeinelike substance; do not mix with caffeine supplements. Kola nut (*Cola spp.*). This African nut contains significant amounts of caffeine. It should not be taken in conjunction with other caffeine-containing products. Maté (*Ilex paraguariensis*). Caffeine is an active ingredient of this South American herb. Do not use it if taking drugs or supplements containing caffeine.
Bear in Mind:	Coffee, tea, chocolate, and cola drinks naturally contain caffeine; it is also added to many soft drinks and "energy boosting" products. Limit your intake of these if you take caffeine supplements. In 1994, two well-conducted studies suggested that postmenopausal women who drink two or more cups of coffee a day and also have a low calcium intake are at greater risk for osteoporosis. Another reputable study in 1997, however, found no connection. Until more is known, postmenopausal women should try to limit caffeine intake and take calcium supplements (1,500 mg daily).

Dovonex

CALCIPOTRIENE

Type of Drug:	Topical antipsoriatic
Description:	Calcipotriene is prescribed to treat psoriasis. It is applied topically (directly to the skin) in the form of a cream, ointment, or solution.
Don't Mix With:	No known herbal interactions.
Bear in Mind:	Calcipotriene can cause your calcium level to rise, which could lead to kidney stones. Drinking lots of liquids (64 ounces a day) may help prevent this. Discuss calcium supplements and your intake of high-calcium foods with your medical practitioner.

Dopar, Larodopa, Lodosyn, Sinemet, Sinemet CR

CARBIDOPA, LEVODOPA

Type of Drug:	Antiparkinsonism
Description:	Levodopa (Dopar, Larodopa) is prescribed for treating Parkinson's disease, restless leg syndrome, and herpes zoster (shingles). Carbidopa (Lodosyn) and the combination of levodopa and carbidopa (Sinemet) are prescribed only for Parkinson's disease. Both carbidopa and levodopa are powerful drugs with numerous serious side effects. They can interact adversely with a number of drugs. Be certain to tell your doctor about any other prescription and nonprescription drugs and dietary supplements you take.
Don't Mix With:	Kava kava (*Piper methysticum*). This relaxant herb may worsen Parkinson's disease symptoms.
Bear in Mind:	Amino acid supplements can temporarily reduce the effectiveness of levodopa. The amino acid tryptophan in the form of 5-HTP could cause tissue changes similar to the disease scleroderma if taken with carbidopa. Do not take amino acid supplements when taking these drugs.
	Your body uses vitamin B6 (pyridoxine) to break down levodopa. Discuss vitamin B6 supplements with your medical practitioner, because taking them may lessen the effectiveness of the drug therapy. High-protein foods can interfere with your absorption of levodopa. Discuss your diet with your medical practitioner.
	Early studies suggest that levodopa depletes your levels of S-adenosyl-l-methionine (SAMe). Taking SAMe supplements, however, could keep the levodopa from working as well. Discuss SAMe supplements with your medical practitioner before you try them.
	Because iron interferes with your absorption of both carbidopa and levodopa, take iron or multivitamin supplements containing iron two hours apart from the drug.

Celebrex

CELECOXIB

Type of Drug:	Cyclooxygenase-2 (COX-2) inhibitor nonsteroidal anti-inflammatory drug (NSAID)
Description:	COX-2 inhibitors are used to treat arthritis. They work by blocking your production of an enzyme that regulates pain and inflammation. COX-2 inhibitors are slightly less likely than are other NSAIDs to cause stomach irritation; they also don't thin your blood.
Don't Mix With:	Salicylate-containing herbs. The herbs meadowsweet (*Filipendula ulmaria*), white willow bark (*Salix alba*), and wintergreen (*Gaultheria procumbens*) contain salicylates. In combination with celecoxib, these herbs could cause severe stomach irritation.
Do Take With:	Milk thistle (*Silybum marianum*). Silymarin, the active compound in the herb milk thistle, may help protect your liver against irritation caused by celecoxib. Consider supplements (150 mg three to four times daily).
Bear in Mind:	Many NSAIDs reduce your absorption of folic acid (folate). Although there is no evidence that celecoxib does this, consider taking supplements (400 mcg daily).

Ceclor, Keflex, Duricef, Suprax, Vantin, others

CEPHALOSPORIN

Type of Drug:	Cephalosporin antibiotic
Description:	Cephalosporin antibiotics are quite similar to penicillin antibiotics. In general, cephalosporin antibiotics kill the bacteria that cause infections and illness. They do not kill viruses, so they are not helpful for colds and flu.
Don't Mix With:	No known herbal interactions.
Bear in Mind:	Cephalosporin antibiotics kill not only the harmful bacteria that cause illness, but also the good bacteria that are normally found in your intestines; this can cause diarrhea. Consider probiotic supplements (at least 1.5 billion live organisms daily, including a mixture of *Lactobacillus acidophilus*, *Bifidobacterium bifidum*, and *Saccharomyces boulardii*).

Allegra, Zyrtec

CETIRIZINE, FEXOFENADINE

Type of Drug:	Antihistamine
Description:	Cetirizine (Zyrtec) and fexofenadine (Allegra) are very similar drugs prescribed to treat the symptoms of seasonal allergies, such as runny nose, sneezing, and itchy eyes. Cetirizine is also used to treat other allergy symptoms such as hives and rashes.
Don't Mix With:	Ephedra (*Ephedra spp.*, also known as ma huang). This stimulant herb can worsen dry mouth, a side effect of both cetirizine and fexofenadine. Similarly avoid the related drugs ephedrine and pseudoephedrine, which are found in many nonprescription cold and allergy remedies.
	Henbane (*Hyascyamus niger*). This herb is toxic and should be used only when prescribed and closely monitored by a qualified practitioner. Because cetirizine and fexofenadine have similar effects to henbane, such as dry mouth, dizziness, and drowsiness, they should never be used in combination with each other.
	Sedative herbs. Sedative herbs may cause excessive drowsiness when combined with cetirizine or fexofenadine. Avoid sedative herbs including chamomile (*Matricaria recutita*), catnip (*Nepeta cataria*), kava kava (*Piper methysticum*), passionflower (*Passiflora incarnata*), St. John's wort (*Hypericum perforatum*), valerian (*Valeriana officinalis*), and others, as well as sedative dietary supplements such as 5-HTP, tryptophan, and SAMe.
Bear in Mind:	Although cetirizine and fexofenadine are less likely than other antihistamines to cause drowsiness and dizziness, these side effects can still occur and are made worse by alcohol. Don't use alcohol when taking these drugs.

CHARCOAL, ACTIVATED CHARCOAL

Type of Drug:	Antidote, adsorbent, laxative
Description:	Activated charcoal is also used for the emergency treatment of some kinds of poisoning. When used alone, activated charcoal helps keep the poison from being absorbed from your stomach into your body. Activated charcoal combined with the sweetener sorbitol is a laxative that helps eliminate the poison from your body. Do not attempt to treat poisoning on your own with activated charcoal. Call for emergency help. Activated charcoal tablets are sometimes used to treat mild diarrhea and intestinal gas.
Don't Mix With:	No known herbal interactions.
Bear in Mind:	Frequent use of activated charcoal tablets can block your absorption of prescription and nonprescription drugs, vitamins, minerals, and other nutrients. Discuss alternative nonprescription remedies with your doctor.

CHLORPHENIRAMINE

Type of Drug:	Antihistamine

Description:

Chlorpheniramine is a nonprescription drug used to treat symptoms of seasonal allergies (sneezing, runny nose, and itchy, watering eyes) and colds and upper respiratory infections (including scratchy throat and nasal congestion). When used in nonprescription allergy and cold formulas, chlorpheniramine is sometimes combined with a decongestant drug such as pseudoephedrine (see page 136). Acetaminophen (see page 57) and dextromethorphan (see page 11) are found in some cold and flu formulas. Decongestant drugs should be avoided by people with diabetes, heart disease, high blood pressure, and many other health problems. Acetaminophen should be avoided by people with liver disease. Read the label carefully.

Don't Mix With:

Ephedra (*Ephedra spp.*, also known as ma huang). This can worsen dry mouth, a side effect of chlorpheniramine. Avoid the related ephedrine and pseudoephedrine, found in cold and allergy remedies. Henbane (*Hyoscyamus niger*). This herb is toxic and should be used only when prescribed and closely monitored by a qualified practitioner. Because chlorpheniramine and henbane have similar side effects (dry mouth, dizziness, and drowsiness), they should never be used together.

Sedative herbs. Sedative herbs may cause excessive drowsiness when combined with chlorpheniramine. Avoid chamomile (*Matricaria recutita*), catnip (*Nepeta cataria*), kava kava (*Piper methysticum*), passionflower (*Passiflora incarnata*), St. John's wort (*Hypericum perforatum*), valerian (*Valeriana officinalis*), and others, as well as sedative dietary supplements such as 5-HTP, tryptophan, and SAMe.

Bear in Mind:

Chlorpheniramine causes drowsiness. Avoid alcohol, which can make the drowsiness worse, and interact adversely with other ingredients in allergy and cold formulas.

Tagamet, Tagamet HB
CIMETIDINE

Type of Drug:	H2 blocker (antacid)
Description:	Cimetidine sharply reduces the production of stomach acid. In prescription form (Tagamet), it is used to treat ulcers and heartburn. In nonprescription form (Tagamet HB), it is used for mild heartburn.
Don't Mix With:	Caffeine-containing herbs. Cimetidine can reduce the rate at which caffeine is eliminated from the body. Use caution if taking caffeine-containing herbs, including guaraná (_Paullinia cupana_), kola nut (_Cola spp._), and maté (_Ilex paraguariensis_), in conjunction with cimetidine as their stimulant effects may last longer.
Do Take With:	Deglycyrrhizinated licorice (DGL, derived from _Glycyrrhiza glabra_). DGL can speed ulcer healing as it stimulates the production of mucus that protects the stomach lining and also has an anti-inflammatory effect. Consider taking supplements (250 mg two to four times daily).
Bear in Mind:	Cimetidine and other H2 blockers reduce the absorption of some vitamins and minerals, including folic acid (folate), vitamin B12 (cobalamin), zinc, and iron. If you use these drugs on a regular basis, consider taking supplements (400 mcg daily of folic acid, 500 mcg daily for vitamin B12, plus a daily multivitamin supplement with minerals). Take them at least two hours apart from cimetidine. Cimetidine may slow the elimination of caffeine. The stimulant effect of coffee, tea, colas, other caffeine-containing soft drinks, and medications containing caffeine (see page 33) may last longer. Magnesium supplements and calcium-, magnesium-, and magnesium/aluminum-based antacids may block the absorption of cimetidine. Take them at least two hours apart from cimetidine.

Cipro

CIPROFLOXACIN

Type of Drug:	Fluoroquinolone antibacterial
Description:	Ciprofloxacin is a widely prescribed member of the fluoroquinolone family of antibacterial drugs. These drugs are used to treat infections against which antibiotics such as penicillin and tetracycline are less effective, such as urinary tract infections and sinus infections. Fluoroquinolones also treat infections in the bones and joints. The asthma drug theophylline can cause a potentially fatal heart arrhythmia if taken with ciprofloxacin. If you use theophylline, be certain to tell your doctor.
Don't Mix With:	Caffeine-containing herbs. Ciprofloxacin can reduce the rate at which the body eliminates caffeine. Exercise caution when combining this drug with caffeine-containing herbs, including guaraná (*Paullinia cupana*), kola nut (*Cola spp.*), and maté (*Ilex paraguariensis*), as their stimulant effects may last longer.
Bear in Mind:	Dairy foods such as milk, yogurt, and cheese interfere with the absorption of ciprofloxacin. Discuss your intake of these foods with your medical practitioner. The minerals calcium, iron, magnesium, and zinc can interfere with the absorption of ciprofloxacin. The reverse is also true: Ciprofloxacin can interfere with the absorption of these minerals. Take mineral supplements, multivitamin supplements with minerals, and calcium- or magnesium-containing antacids, two hours apart from ciprofloxacin. Ciprofloxacin may slow down the elimination of caffeine. The stimulant effect of coffee, tea, colas, other caffeine-containing soft drinks, and drugs containing caffeine, may last longer; use caution if consuming caffeine-containing substances when taking ciprofloxacin.

Platinol, Platinol-AQ
CISPLATIN

Type of Drug:	Anticancer (antineoplastic)
Description:	Cisplatin is an anticancer drug used primarily to treat cancer of the bladder, ovaries, and testicles, but is also used to treat many other kinds of cancer. Cisplatin is a very powerful drug that can interact adversely with other drugs. Be sure to discuss any other prescription and nonprescription drugs and dietary supplements you take, including those suggested here, with your medical practitioner.
Don't Mix With:	No known herbal interactions.
Do Take With:	Milk thistle (*Silybum marianum*). In animal studies, milk thistle, which contains the active compound silymarin, helps protect against liver damage from cisplatin. Although there are no human studies yet, many scientists believe milk thistle can be helpful. Discuss supplements with your medical practitioner (150 mg three to four times daily).
	Natural nausea remedies. Ginger (*Zingiber officinale*) capsules and the homeopathic remedy nux vomica 30C (once a day or as directed by your medical practitioner) may help relieve nausea and vomiting, which are common side effects of cisplatin.
Bear in Mind:	Cisplatin can deplete the body's stores of calcium, magnesium, phosphate, potassium, and sodium. Discuss iron-free multivitamin and mineral supplements with your medical practitioner. Preliminary studies suggest that injections of glutathione, the body's most abundant natural antioxidant, can help relieve some of the side effects of cisplatin. N-acetyl cysteine (also called NAC) and selenium supplements can also help increase the glutathione level. Discuss this with your medical practitioner and consider taking supplements (NAC, 600 mg three times daily; selenium, 200 mcg daily).

Biaxin

CLARITHROMYCIN

Type of Drug:	Macrolide antibiotic
Description:	Clarithromycin is used to treat bacterial infections. It is often prescribed for respiratory tract infections, ulcers, and skin infections. This drug has numerous interactions with other prescription drugs. Be certain to tell your doctor about any other prescription and nonprescription drugs and dietary supplements you take. If you take any statin drug such as lovastatin (see page 103) or atorvastatin (see page 24), do not take clarithromycin. The combination could cause a potentially fatal muscle disease.
Don't Mix With:	Digitalis (*Digitalis spp.*, also known as foxglove). Clarithromycin can raise the level of both the dangerous herb digitalis and digoxin, a drug with similar effects. Do not mix the two.
Bear in Mind:	Clarithromycin kills not only the harmful bacteria that cause illness but also the good bacteria that are normally found in your intestines. This can cause diarrhea. Consider taking probiotic supplements (at least 1.5 billion live organisms daily, including a mixture of *Lactobacillus acidophilus*, *Bifidobacterium bifidum*, and *Saccharomyces boulardii*).

Antihist-l, Tavist, Tavist-D

CLEMASTINE

Type of Drug:	Antihistamine
Description:	Clemastine is a nonprescription drug used to treat symptoms of seasonal allergies, including sneezing, runny nose, and itchy and watering eyes. In combination with phenylpropanolamine (see page 127), clemastine (Tavist-D) is used to treat the symptoms of colds and upper respiratory infections, including scratchy throat and nasal congestion.
Don't Mix With: 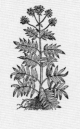	Ephedra (*Ephedra spp.*, also known as ma huang). This stimulant herb can worsen dry mouth, a side effect of clemastine. Similarly, avoid the related drugs ephedrine and pseudoephedrine, which are found in many nonprescription cold and allergy remedies. Henbane (*Hyoscyamus niger*). This herb is toxic and should be used only when prescribed and closely monitored by a licensed practitioner. Because both clemastine and henbane have similar side effects, such as dry mouth, dizziness, and drowsiness, they should never be used in combination with each other. Sedative herbs. When combined with clemastine, sedative herbs may cause excessive drowsiness. Avoid sedative herbs such as chamomile (*Matricaria recutita*), catnip (*Nepeta cataria*), kava kava (*Piper methysticum*), passionflower (*Passiflora incarnata*), St. John's wort (*Hypericum perforatum*), valerian (*Valeriana officinalis*), and others, as well as sedative dietary supplements such as 5-HTP, tryptophan, and SAMe.
Bear in Mind:	Clemastine causes drowsiness and difficulty concentrating. Because alcohol can make these side effects worse, do not use it in conjunction with this drug.

Cleocin

CLINDAMYCIN

Type of Drug:	Antibiotic
Description:	Clindamycin is prescribed to treat bacterial infections, including vaginal infections, lung abscesses, infected wounds, and abdominal infections. It is also used topically to treat acne and rosacea. When taken orally, clindamycin is a very powerful drug that can cause colitis, a severe intestinal irritation.
Don't Mix With:	No known herbal interactions.
Bear in Mind:	Clindamycin kills not only the harmful bacteria that cause illness, but also the good bacteria that are normally found in your intestines; this can cause diarrhea. Consider probiotic supplements (at least 1.5 billion live organisms daily, including a mixture of *Lactobacillus acidophilus*, *Bifidobacterium bifidum*, and *Saccharomyces boulardii*).

Atromid-S
CLOFIBRATE

Type of Drug:	Antihyperlipidemic
Description:	Clofibrate is prescribed primarily for people who have high triglyceride (a type of fat present in the blood) levels. It is also sometimes prescribed to reduce high cholesterol levels. Clofibrate can interact adversely with a number of drugs, especially blood thinners, statin drugs, and drugs used to treat diabetes. It can also cause liver damage and gallstones. Be certain to tell your doctor about any other prescription and nonprescription drugs and dietary supplements you take. Because of the risk of side effects and interactions, clofibrate is used only when other, safer drugs haven't helped.
Don't Mix With:	No known herbal interactions.
Do Take With:	Milk thistle (*Silybum marianum*). Silymarin, the active compound in the herb milk thistle, may help protect your liver against damage from clofibrate. Consider taking supplements (150 mg three to four times daily).
Bear in Mind:	Clofibrate may reduce your absorption of Vitamin B12. Consider taking supplements (500 mcg daily, taken at least two hours apart from the drug). To avoid stomach upset, take clofibrate with food or milk.

Anafranil

CLOMIPRAMINE

Type of Drug:	Tricyclic antidepressant
Description:	Clomipramine is used to treat depression. Like other tricyclic antidepressants, it works by affecting the way chemicals called neurotransmitters, including serotonin and norepinephrine, move in and out of your nerve endings.
Don't Mix With:	Ephedra (*Ephedra spp.*, also known as ma huang). Taking ephedra with any tricyclic antidepressant raises your risk of serious high blood pressure and heart arrhythmias. Similarly, avoid the related drugs ephedrine and pseudoephedrine, which are found in many nonprescription cold and allergy remedies.

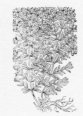

Sedative herbs. Sedative herbs may cause excessive drowsiness when combined with clomipramine. Avoid sedative herbs such as chamomile (*Matricaria recutita*), catnip (*Nepeta cataria*), kava kava (*Piper methysticum*), passionflower (*Passiflora incarnata*), St. John's wort (*Hypericum perforatum*), valerian (*Valeriana officinalis*), and others, as well as sedative dietary supplements such as 5-HTP, tryptophan, and SAMe.

St. John's wort (*Hypericum perforatum*). Research suggests that this herb and clomipramine work in similar ways. Until more is known, don't take clomipramine in conjunction with St. John's wort.

Yohimbe. (*Pausinystalia yohimbe*) This dangerous herb is said to improve male sexual function. Don't use this herb when taking clomipramine; the combination may cause a dangerous rise in blood pressure.

Bear in Mind:	Heart problems can be a side effect of tricyclic antidepressants, possibly because these drugs lower your production of coenzyme Q10 (CoQ10 or ubiquinone). Coenzyme is needed to produce energy in your cells, including the cells of your heart. Consider taking supplements (20 to 50 mg daily).

Catapres

CLONIDINE

Type of Drug:	Antihypertensive
Description:	Clonidine is prescribed for lowering high blood pressure. It is also sometimes prescribed to help people withdraw from addiction to alcohol and other substances, including tobacco.
Don't Mix With:	Blood vessel relaxing herbs. *Coleus forskohlii*, garlic (*Allium sativum*), ginkgo (*Ginkgo biloba*), and hawthorn (*Crataegus monogyna*) relax your blood vessels and are sometimes used to treat high blood pressure. Although there have been no studies, it's possible that combining these herbs with clonidine could make your blood pressure drop too low.
	Licorice (*Glycyrrhiza glabra*). Glycyrrhizin, a compound naturally occurring in licorice, can cause an increase in blood pressure. If you are taking clonidine to lower blood pressure, avoid this herb unless it is deglycyrrhizinated licorice (DGL).
	Yohimbe (*Pausinystalia yohimbe*). This dangerous herb is sometimes used for erectile dysfunction; one of its side effects is a sharp rise in blood pressure. Never mix it with clonidine – dangerous changes in your blood pressure could occur.
Bear in Mind:	Clonidine has a depressive effect; so does alcohol. Don't use alcohol when taking this drug.
	Clonidine may reduce the bioavailability of coenzyme Q10 (CoQ10 or ubiquinone), which is needed for energy production within your cells. Consider taking supplements (20-50 mg daily).
	Vitamin E can increase blood pressure in certain susceptible people, according to some studies. Consult your doctor before taking vitamin E supplements if you have high blood pressure.

Empirin, Phenergan, Robitussin AC, others

CODEINE

Type of Drug:	Narcotic analgesic
Description:	Codeine is a powerful narcotic pain reliever used by itself or combined with a nonsteroidal anti-inflammatory drug such as aspirin (see page 22) or acetaminophen (see page 11). Codeine is also used as a prescription cough suppressant by itself or in combination with other drugs (Phenergan, Robitussin AC).

Don't Mix With:

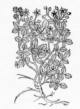

Tannin-containing herbs. Herbs that are high in tannin, including black walnut (*Juglans nigra*), red raspberry (*Rubus idaeus*), oak (*Quercus spp.*), uva ursi (*Arctostaphylos uva ursi*), and witch hazel (*Hamamelis virginiana*), can interfere with your absorption of codeine, as can the tannins in tea. Don't consume these substances within two hours of taking this drug.

Bear in Mind:

Codeine causes drowsiness, impaired judgment, and loss of coordination. Alcohol makes these side effects worse. Don't use alcohol in conjunction with this drug.

Constipation is a common side effect of codeine. To lessen this problem, eat plenty of high-fiber foods, such as fresh fruits and vegetables and whole grains, and drink 64 ounces of water daily.

This drug is sold only in generic form.

COLCHICINE

Type of Drug:	Antigout
Description:	Colchicine relieves pain and inflammation in people with gout. It is also used long-term to prevent gout attacks. Colchicine is a good example of a traditional herbal remedy that has become a standard drug. The original source of this drug is a type of crocus called *Colchicum autumnale*.
Don't Mix With: 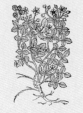	Tannin-containing herbs. Herbs that are high in tannin, including black walnut (*Juglans nigra*), red raspberry (*Rubus idaeus*), oak (*Quercus spp.*), uva ursi (*Arctostaphylos uva ursi*), and witch hazel (*Hamamelis virginiana*), can interfere with your absorption of colchicine, as can the tannins in tea. Don't consume these substances within two hours of taking this drug.
Bear in Mind:	Colchicine may make you much more sensitive to alcohol. Because alcohol is also not recommended for people suffering from gout, avoid it when taking this drug. Colchicine may block your absorption of vitamin B12 (cobalamin). If you use this drug on a regular basis, consider taking supplements (500 mcg daily). Colchicine may also block your absorption of beta carotene, which your body uses to produce vitamin A. Consider taking supplements of mixed carotenes (25,000 IU daily).

Cenestin, Premarin, Premphase, Prempro

CONJUGATED ESTROGEN

Type of Drug:	Estrogen/progesterone hormone replacement
Description:	Conjugated estrogens combine several different estrogen-like hormones into one medication (Premarin, Cenestin). Conjugated estrogens are often combined with a semisynthetic compound called medroxyprogesterone (Prempro, Premphase). These drugs are prescribed to treat the symptoms of menopause, including hot flashes and vaginal dryness, and to help prevent osteoporosis in women.
Don't Mix With:	Black cohosh (*Cimicifuga racemosa*). Black cohosh contains phytoestrogens, plant hormones similar to human estrogen. Combining it with prescription estrogen drugs could raise your estrogen level too high.
	Chaste tree (*Vitex agnus-castus*). Chaste tree affects your levels of the hormone prolactin, which in turn can affect your natural production of estrogen and how your body uses supplemental estrogen.
	Other estrogenic herbs. The herbs dong quai (*Angelica sinensis*) and red clover (*Trifolium pratense*) may have estrogen-like effects. Laboratory studies have shown that the herbs licorice (*Glycyrrhiza glabra*), thyme (*Thymus spp.*), turmeric (*Curcuma longa*), hops (*Humulus lupulus*), and vervain (*Verbena spp.*) may also modulate estrogen activity. Discuss the use of these herbs with your medical practitioner before using them.
Bear in Mind:	Studies have shown that soy isoflavones (estrogen-like substances) can help to relieve menopause symptoms. Ipriflavone, a type of soy isoflavone, can help prevent osteoporosis. Combining soy isoflavones with prescription estrogen drugs could raise your estrogen levels too high. If you want to use soy isoflavones in combination with or instead of supplemental estrogen, discuss it with your doctor first.

Cytoxan, Neosar

CYCLOPHOSPHAMIDE

Type of Drug:	Anticancer
Description:	Cyclophosphamide is a drug used in chemotherapy for various types of cancer. It is a powerful drug that can have severe side effects and interact adversely with a number of other drugs. Be certain to tell your doctor about any other prescription and nonprescription drugs and dietary supplements you take.
Don't Mix With:	Antioxidant herbs. In theory, herbs with high antioxidant activity could reduce the effectiveness of cyclophosphamide. Until more is known, avoid herbs such as ginkgo (*Ginkgo biloba*), lemon balm (*Melissa officinalis*), mints (*Mentha spp.*), oregano (*Origanum vulgare*), rosemary (*Rosmarinus officinalis*), thyme (*Thymus spp.*), and turmeric (*Curcuma longa*). Also avoid grapeseed and pine bark extract, including Pycnogenol® because of their antioxidant properties.
Do Take With:	Natural nausea remedies. Ginger (*Zingiber officinale*) capsules or tea and the homeopathic remedy nux vomica 30C may help relieve nausea and vomiting, common side effects of cyclophosphamide. Discuss these remedies and dosage recommendations with your medical practitioner before trying them. Turkey tail (*Coriolus versicolor*). Called yun zhi in Chinese and kawaratake in Japanese, turkey tail is a type of mushroom. A substance in turkey tail called PSK may help protect the immune system from the damaging effects of chemotherapy drugs such as cyclophosphamide. Discuss turkey tail with your doctor and consider taking supplements (625 mg one to two times daily).
Bear in Mind:	Although there are no studies, it is possible that the antioxidant vitamins A, beta carotene, C, and E could reduce the effectiveness of cyclophosamide. Other studies suggest that these vitamins might be helpful. Discuss vitamin supplements with your doctor.

Neoral, Sandimmune

CYCLOSPORINE

Type of Drug:	Immunosuppressant
Description:	Cyclosporine suppresses your immune system and prevents rejection of transplanted organs. This very powerful drug is also sometimes used to treat other serious conditions, including aplastic anemia, ulcerative colitis, multiple sclerosis, and severe psoriasis. Cyclosporine has several serious side effects and interacts adversely with a number of drugs. Be certain to tell your doctor about any other prescription and nonprescription drugs and dietary supplements you take. Cyclosporine is usually used along with corticosteroid drugs such as prednisone (see page 131).
Don't Mix With:	St. John's wort (*Hypericum perforatum*). This herb significantly lowers the amount of cyclosporine you absorb, to the point where organ rejection might occur. Don't use this herb if taking cyclosporine.
Bear in Mind:	A substance in grapefruit or grapefruit juice may reduce the rate of elimination of cyclosporine. This can increase the amount of cyclosporine in your body to dangerous levels. Avoid grapefruit and grapefruit juice when taking this drug. Cyclosporine increases the amount of potassium in your blood. Don't use potassium supplements or salt substitutes when taking this drug. One study in 1996 showed that water-soluble vitamin E may be helpful for improving your absorption of cyclosporine. Discuss taking vitamin E supplements with your doctor – do not start taking them on your own.

Norpramin

DESIPRAMINE

Type of Drug:	Tricyclic antidepressant
Description:	Desipramine is used to treat depression. Like the other tricyclic antidepressants, it works by affecting the way chemicals called neurotransmitters, including serotonin and norepinephrine, move in and out of your nerve endings.

Don't Mix With:

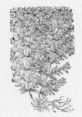

Ephedra (*Ephedra spp.*, also known as ma huang). Taking ephedra with any tricyclic antidepressant raises your risk of serious high blood pressure and heart arrhythmias. Similarly, avoid the related drugs ephedrine and pseudoephedrine, which are found in many nonprescription cold and allergy remedies.

Sedative herbs. Sedative herbs may cause excessive drowsiness when combined with desipramine. Avoid sedative herbs such as chamomile (*Matricaria recutita*), catnip (*Nepeta cataria*), kava kava (*Piper methysticum*), passionflower (*Passiflora incarnata*), St. John's wort (*Hypericum perforatum*), valerian (*Valeriana officinalis*), and others, as well as sedative dietary supplements such as 5-HTP, tryptophan, and SAMe.

St. John's wort (*Hypericum perforatum*). Research suggests that this herb and desipramine work in similar ways. Until more is known, don't take desipramine in conjunction with St. John's wort.

Yohimbe (*Pausinystalia yohimbe*). This dangerous herb is said to improve male sexual function. Don't use this herb when taking desipramine; the combination may cause a dangerous rise in blood pressure.

Bear in Mind: Heart problems can be a side effect of tricyclic antidepressants, possibly because these drugs lower your production of coenzyme Q10 (CoQ10 or ubiquinone). Coenzyme Q10 is needed to produce energy in your cells, including the cells of your heart. Consider taking supplements (20 to 50 mg daily).

Decadron, Dexone, Hexadrol

DEXAMETHASONE

Type of Drug:	Corticosteroid
Description:	These synthetic hormones are used to treat a wide variety of severe disorders, particularly those that involve inflammation, including arthritis, psoriasis, allergies, asthma, and inflammatory bowel disease. They are also used to treat autoimmune diseases such as lupus erythematosus and transplant rejection. Corticosteroids are powerful drugs that can cause serious side effects and interact adversely with a wide range of drugs. Tell your doctor about any other prescription and nonprescription drugs and dietary supplements you take.
Don't Mix With:	Digitalis (*Digitalis spp.*, also known as foxglove). This dangerous herb is very similar to the heart drug digoxin (see page 61), which may worsen the side effects of dexamethasone. Do not use either digitalis or digoxin if taking this drug. Ephedra (*Ephedra spp.*, also known as ma huang). The herb ephedra naturally contains ephedrine, which can reduce the effectiveness of corticosteroids. Do not use it when taking dexamethasone. Similarly, avoid ephedrine (see page 71) and pseudoephedrine (see page 136), which are found in many nonprescription cold and allergy remedies.
Bear in Mind:	Corticosteroids can make you retain sodium, found in salt. Discuss reducing your salt intake with your doctor. Long-term use of corticosteroids can interfere with your body's absorption of calcium, which may lead to osteoporosis. Consider taking supplements (1,000 mg calcium daily, 400 IU vitamin D daily). Corticosteroids may also reduce your level of vitamin B6 (pyridoxine). Consider supplements (50 mg daily). Long-term use of corticosteroids may deplete your levels of magnesium. Consider supplements (300–400 mg daily). Long-term use of corticosteroids can contribute to the development of diabetes. Consider a chromium picolinate supplement (200 mcg daily).

Benylin DM, Robitussin, others

DEXTROMETHORPHAN

Type of Drug:	Cough suppressant
Description:	Dextromethorphan helps stop coughing from colds, flu, upper respiratory infections, and allergies. It is found in many nonprescription cough formulas, either by itself (Benylin DM,) or in combination with other cough medicines and decongestants (Robitussin).
Don't Mix With:	Sedative herbs. When combined with dextromethorphan, these herbs may cause excessive drowsiness. Avoid sedative herbs such as chamomile (*Matricaria recutita*), catnip (*Nepeta cataria*), kava kava (*Piper methysticum*), passionflower (*Passiflora incarnata*), St. John's wort (*Hypericum perforatum*), valerian (*Valeriana officinalis*), and others, as well as sedative dietary supplements such as 5-HTP, tryptophan, and SAMe.
Bear in Mind:	Dextromethorphan can cause drowsiness. Alcohol makes this side effect worse; it should be avoided when taking this drug.

Valium

DIAZEPAM

Type of Drug:	Antianxiety
Description:	Diazepam, along with other members of the benzodiazepine family such as alprazolam (Xanax) and chlordiazepoxide (Librium) is prescribed to relieve anxiety and tension; it is also used as a muscle relaxant. Benzodiazepine drugs are safe and effective and have few side effects, but they are potentially addictive.
Don't Mix With:	Digitalis (*Digitalis spp.*, also known as foxglove). This dangerous herb is very similar to the heart drug digoxin (see page 61). Diazepam raises the level of digoxin in your blood. Don't take digitalis if you are taking diazepam.
	Sedative herbs. When combined with diazepam, these herbs may cause excessive drowsiness. Avoid sedative herbs such as chamomile (*Matricaria recutita*), catnip (*Nepeta cataria*), kava kava (*Piper methysticum*), passionflower (Passiflora incarnata), St. John's wort (*Hypericum perforatum*), valerian (*Valeriana officinalis*), and others, as well as sedative dietary supplements such as 5-HTP, tryptophan, and SAMe.
Bear in Mind:	Diazepam depresses your central nervous system, as does alcohol. Mixing the two may cause excessive drowsiness and potentially fatal breathing difficulties.
	Don't take macrolide antibiotics, such as azithromycin (see page 26), clarithromycin (see page 44), erythromycin (see page 73), and others with any benzodiazepine drug. These drugs can raise your level of the benzodiazepine drug dangerously high.

Bemote, Byclomine, Di Spaz, others

DICYCLOMINE

Type of Drug:	Antispasmodic
Description:	Dicyclomine is prescribed for irritable bowel syndrome and related digestive problems.
Don't Mix With:	No known herbal interactions.
Bear in Mind:	A side effect of dicyclomine is a reduction in your ability to sweat. Avoid overheating. Another side effect of dicyclomine is constipation. To lessen this problem, eat plenty of high-fiber foods, such as fresh fruits and vegetables and whole grains, and drink 64 ounces of water daily. You may also want to discuss remedies with your doctor.

Videx

DIDANOSINE

Type of Drug:	Antiviral
Description:	Didanosine is used in combination with AZT (see page 27) and the protease inhibitor indinavir (see page 91) as part of a "cocktail" of drugs to treat HIV infection and AIDS. Didanosine is a very powerful drug that can have a number of extremely serious side effects. It can also interact badly with a number of other drugs. Be certain to tell your doctor about any other prescription and nonprescription drugs and dietary supplements you take.
Don't Mix With:	No known herbal interactions.
Do Take With:	Lentinan, a complex sugar found in shiitake mushrooms, may help didanosine work better. Lentinan must be given by injection; eating a lot of shiitake mushrooms will not have any effect. Discuss this supplement with your medical practitioner. Milk thistle (*Silybum marianum*). Silymarin, the active compound in the herb milk thistle, may help protect your liver against damage from didanosine. Consider taking supplements (200 mg daily).

Lanoxin

DIGOXIN

Type of Drug:	Digitalis glycoside
Description:	Digoxin (Lanoxin) and the related drug digitoxin (Crystodigin) are prescribed to treat congestive heart failure and other heart conditions that make your heart beat very rapidly, such as tachycardia.

Don't Mix With:

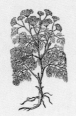

Digitalis (*Digitalis spp.*, also known as foxglove). This dangerous herb acts in ways very similar to digoxin. Never combine the two – a potentially fatal increase in your digoxin level will occur.

Herbal diuretics. If you are taking a prescription diuretic do not take nonprescription or herbal diuretics including bilberry leaf (*Vaccinium myrtillus*), burdock (*Arctium lappa*), damiana (*Turnera diffusa*), dandelion (*Taraxacum officinale*), fennel seed (*Foeniculum vulgare*), goldenrod (*Solidago virgaurea*), horsetail (*Equisetum arvense*), kava kava (*Piper methysticum*), kola nut (*Cola spp.*), marshmallow (*Althaea officinalis*), maté (*Ilex paraguariensis*), parsley (*Petroselinum spp.*), sarsaparilla (*Smilax spp.*), saw palmetto (*Serenoa repens*), uva ursi (*Arctostaphylos uva ursi*), vervain (*Verbena spp.*), and yarrow (*Achillea millefolium*).

Hawthorn (*Crataegus spp.*). The herb hawthorn is often used to treat mild congestive heart failure. Combining the two may cause problems as they both are used to treat the same condition and may have additive effects.

Herbal laxatives. Using herbal laxatives such as cascara sagrada (*Rhamnus purshiana*) and senna (*Senna alexandrina*) can decrease the level of digoxin in your blood and can also deplete your potassium level. Don't use them if taking this drug.

Licorice (*Glycyrrhiza glabra*). Large amounts of licorice can reduce your potassium level. Since digoxin also reduces potassium levels, do not combine the two as it may make your potassium level dangerously low. This effect does not occur as readily with deglycyrrhizinated licorice (DGL) or with artificial licorice flavoring.

Cardizem, Dilacor, Tiamate, Tiazac, others

DILTIAZEM

Type of Drug:	Calcium channel blocker
Description:	Diltiazem is prescribed for high blood pressure, angina, and to help prevent a second heart attack. Diltiazem is a calcium channel blocker, a drug that causes blood vessels to relax and widen.
Don't Mix With:	No known herbal interactions.
Do Take With:	Milk thistle (Silybum marianum). Silymarin, the active substance in the herb milk thistle, may help protect against liver damage from diltiazem. Consider taking supplements (200 mg daily).
Bear in Mind:	A substance in grapefruit or grapefruit juice may reduce the rate of excretion of other calcium channel blocker drugs such as felodipine and nifedipine (see page 112). This can cause a dangerous increase in the amount of these drugs in your blood. Although there have been no reports of a similar effect with diltiazem, until more is known, don't eat grapefruit or drink grapefruit juice if you take any calcium channel blocker.

Dimetabs, Dramamine, Marmine, Nico-Vert, Triptone, others

DIMENHYDRINATE

Type of Drug:	Antihistamine and antiemetic (drug that relieves nausea and vomiting)
Description:	Dimenhydrinate is used to treat and prevent nausea, vomiting, and dizziness from motion sickness. This drug is a combination of two drugs, diphenhydramine (see page 64) and chlorotheophylline.
Don't Mix With:	Henbane (*Hyoscyamus niger*). This herb is toxic and should be used only when prescribed and closely monitored by a qualified practitioner. Because both dimenhydrinate and henbane have similar side effects, such as dry mouth, dizziness and drowsiness, they should never be used in combination with each other. Sedative herbs. When combined with dimenhydrinate, these herbs may cause excessive drowsiness. Avoid sedative herbs such as chamomile (*Matricaria recutita*), catnip (*Nepeta cataria*), kava kava (*Piper methysticum*), passionflower (*Passiflora incarnata*), St. John's wort (*Hypericum perforatum*), valerian (*Valeriana officinalis*), and others, as well as sedative dietary supplements such as 5-HTP, tryptophan, and SAMe.
Bear in Mind:	Dimenhydrinate causes drowsiness. Alcohol makes this effect worse; do not use it if taking this drug.

Anacin PM, Benadryl, Benylin, Excedrin PM, Nytol, Sleep-Eze, Sominex, Tylenol PM

DIPHENHYDRAMINE

Type of Drug:	Antihistamine

Description: Diphenhydramine is an antihistamine used to treat the symptoms of seasonal allergies, such as runny nose, itchy eyes, and scratchy throat, and to relieve other allergy symptoms such as rashes and hives (Benadryl, Benylin). Diphenhydramine is used in nonprescription sleep aids either by itself (Nytol, Sleep-Eze, Sominex) or in combination with other ingredients (Anacin PM, Excedrin PM, Tylenol PM).

Don't Mix With: Henbane (*Hyoscyamus niger*). This herb is toxic and should be used only when prescribed and closely monitored by a qualified practitioner. Because diphenhydramine and henbane have similar side effects, such as dry mouth, dizziness, and drowsiness, they should never be used in combination with each other.

Sedative herbs. When combined with diphenhydramine, these herbs may cause excessive drowsiness. Avoid sedative herbs such as chamomile (*Matricaria recutita*), catnip (*Nepeta cataria*), kava kava (*Piper methysticum*), passionflower (*Passiflora incarnata*), St. John's wort (*Hypericum perforatum*), valerian (*Valeriana officinalis*), and others, as well as sedative dietary supplements such as 5-HTP, tryptophan, and SAMe.

Bear in Mind: Diphenhydramine causes drowsiness. Alcohol makes this effect worse; do not use it if taking this drug.

The hormone melatonin is used as a natural sleep aid. Because little is known about possible drug interactions, don't combine it with diphenhydramine or any other prescription or nonprescription sleep aids. To do so may make you dangerously drowsy.

Antabuse

DISULFIRAM

Type of Drug:	Alcohol abuse deterrent
Description:	Disulfiram is prescribed to help people avoid drinking alcohol. The drug causes a very unpleasant reaction, including headache, nausea, vomiting, sweating, and dizziness, when the patient drinks or comes into physical contact with even a very small amount of alcohol.
Don't Mix With: 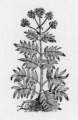	Sedative herbs. When combined with disulfiram, these herbs may cause excessive drowsiness. Avoid sedative herbs such as chamomile (*Matricaria recutita*), catnip (*Nepeta cataria*), kava kava (*Piper methysticum*), passionflower (*Passiflora incarnata*), St. John's wort (*Hypericum perforatum*), valerian (*Valeriana officinalis*), and others, as well as sedative dietary supplements such as 5-HTP, tryptophan, and SAMe. Caffeine-containing herbs. Disulfiram, in combination with caffeine, may cause excessive stimulation. Avoid the herbs guaraná (*Paullinia cupana*), kola nut (*Cola spp.*), and maté (*Ilex paraguariensis*) as they all contain caffeine.
Bear in Mind:	Avoid alcohol in any form, even aftershaves and perfumes and the fumes from alcohol-containing chemicals such as paint thinner. Read the ingredients label on all products carefully. Avoid elixir or liquid cough, cold, flu, and diarrhea remedies that contain alcohol. Avoid mouthwashes and gargles. Avoid vinegar and any food or sauce that may contain alcohol. Coffee, tea, chocolate, and cola drinks naturally contain caffeine; it is also added to many soft drinks and "energy-boosting" products. Avoid these products if you take disulfiram.

Sinequan

DOXEPIN

Type of Drug:	Tricyclic antidepressant
Description:	Doxepin is used to treat depression. Like other tricyclic antidepressants, it works by affecting the way chemicals called neurotransmitters, including serotonin and norepinephrine, move in and out of your nerve endings.
Don't Mix With:	Ephedra (*Ephedra spp.*, also known as ma huang). Taking ephedra with any tricyclic antidepressant raises your risk of serious high blood pressure and heart arrhythmias. Similarly, avoid the related drugs ephedrine and pseudoephedrine, which are found in many nonprescription cold and allergy remedies.
	Sedative herbs. Sedative drugs may cause excessive drowsiness when combined with doxepin. Avoid sedative herbs such as chamomile (*Matricaria recutita*), catnip (*Nepeta cataria*), kava kava (*Piper methysticum*), passionflower (*Passiflora incarnata*), St. John's wort (*Hypericum perforatum*), valerian (*Valeriana officinalis*), and others, as well as sedative dietary supplements such as 5-HTP, tryptophan, and SAMe.
	St. John's wort (*Hypericum perforatum*). Research suggests that this herb and doxepin work in similar ways. Until more is known, don't take it in conjunction with St. John's wort.
	Yohimbe. (*Pausinystalia yohimbe*) This dangerous herb is said to improve male sexual function. Don't use this herb when taking doxepin; the combination may cause a dangerous rise in blood pressure.
Bear in Mind:	Heart problems can be a side effect of tricyclic antidepressants, possibly because these drugs lower your production of coenzyme Q10 (CoQ10 or ubiquinone). Coenzyme Q10 is needed to produce energy in your cells, including the cells of the heart. Consider taking supplements (20 to 50 mg daily).

Adriamycin, Rubex

DOXORUBICIN

Type of Drug:	Anticancer
Description:	Doxorubicin is a very toxic drug used to treat many types of cancer. Because doxorubicin works by interfering with the growth not only of cancer cells but also of normal cells, this drug has many serious side effects, including heart problems. Be sure to discuss any prescription or nonprescription drugs and dietary supplements you are taking with your medical practitioner.
Don't Mix With:	No known herbal interactions.
Bear in Mind:	The risk of heart damage from doxorubicin may be lowered if you take coenzyme Q10 (CoQ10 or ubiquinone) before treatments. Animal studies have shown that vitamins C and E may also have a protective effect. Discuss this with your doctor and consider taking supplements (30–100 mg coenzyme Q10 daily, 1000 mg vitamin C daily, 400 IU vitamin E daily). Doxorubicin can increase your risk of kidney stones. Drinking at least 64 ounces of fluids daily can help prevent this.

Doryx, Monodox, Vibramycin, others

DOXYCYCLINE

Type of Drug:	Tetracycline antibiotic
Description:	Doxycycline is prescribed for bacterial infections. It is often prescribed to prevent or treat traveler's diarrhea.
Don't Mix With:	Berberine-containing herbs. Goldenseal (*Hydrastis canadensis*), barberry (*Berberis vulgaris*), and Oregon grape (*Mahonia aquifolium* contain berberine, an antibacterial chemical. It is possible that berberine interferes with the your absorption of tetracycline, a drug very similar to doxycycline. Until more is known, don't use these herbs when taking doxycycline.
Bear in Mind:	The calcium in milk and dairy products can interfere with the absorption of doxycycline. Discuss your intake of these foods with your medical practitioner.
	The aluminum, calcium, and magnesium in antacids can interfere with your absorption of doxycycline, as can the calcium, iron, magnesium, zinc, and other minerals in supplements and multivitamins with minerals. Take these antacids and supplements two hours apart from this drug.
	Doxycycline kills not only the harmful bacteria that cause illness but also the good bacteria that are normally found in your intestines; this can cause diarrhea. Consider taking probiotic supplements (at least 1.5 billion live organisms daily, including a mixture of *Lactobacillus acidophilus*, *Bifidobacterium bifidum*, and *Saccharomyces boulardii*).

Unisom

DOXYLAMINE

Type of Drug:	Antihistamine
Description:	Doxylamine is an antihistamine, a type of drug usually used to treat allergies, but it is used primarily as a nonprescription sleep aid, either by itself (Unisom) or as an ingredient in nighttime cold formulas.
Don't Mix With:	Henbane (*Hyoscyamus niger*). This herb is toxic and should be used only when prescribed and closely monitored by a qualified practitioner. Because both doxylamine and henbane have similar side effects, such as dry mouth, dizziness, and drowsiness, they should never be used in combination with each other. Sedative herbs. When combined with doxylamine, these herbs may cause excessive drowsiness. Avoid sedative herbs such as chamomile (*Matricaria recutita*), catnip (*Nepeta cataria*), kava kava (*Piper methysticum*), passionflower (*Passiflora incarnata*), St. John's wort (*Hypericum perforatum*), valerian (*Valeriana officinalis*), and others, as well as sedative dietary supplements such as 5-HTP, tryptophan, and SAMe.
Bear in Mind:	Doxylamine causes drowsiness. Alcohol makes this effect worse. Do not use alcohol in conjunction with this drug. The hormone melatonin is used as a natural sleep aid. Don't combine it with doxylamine or any other prescription or nonprescription sleep aid. To do so may cause dangerous drowsiness.

Spectazole

ECANAZOLE

Type of Drug:	Antifungal
Description:	Spectazole is an antifungal cream prescribed for fungal infections of the skin, including athlete's foot, jock itch, and ringworm.
Don't Mix With:	No known herbal interactions.
Do Take With:	Echinacea (*Echinacea* spp). According to one study, women who took the herb echinacea while using econazole cream had fewer recurrences of vaginal yeast infections compared to women who used the cream alone. Consider taking supplements (500 mg three times daily until infection resolves).

Bronkaid, Pretz-D, Primatene, Vicks Vatronol, others

EPHEDRINE

Type of Drug:	Bronchodilator and decongestant
Description:	In prescription and nonprescription forms, ephedrine is used to relieve asthma (Bronkaid, Primatene, others). As a nasal spray (Pretz-D) or in drops (Vicks Vatronol), it is used to treat nasal congestion. If you have asthma, discuss ephedrine products with your doctor before you try them.
Don't Mix With:	Caffeine-containing herbs. The stimulant effect of caffeine can make the side effects of ephedrine, such as nervousness, restlessness, insomnia, and dizziness, worse. Avoid caffeine-containing herbs, including guaraná (*Paullinia cupana*), kola nut (*Cola spp.*), and maté (*Ilex paraguariensis*). Ephedra (*Ephedra spp.*, also known as ma huang). Ephedrine was originally isolated from ephedra. Taking ephedra with any product containing ephedrine could increase the side effects of the drug, including nervousness, insomnia, dizziness, high blood pressure, and heart arrhythmias. Tannin-containing herbs. Herbs that are high in tannin, including black walnut (*Juglans nigra*), red raspberry (*Rubus idaeus*), oak (*Quercus spp.*), uva ursi (*Arctostaphylos uva ursi*), and witch hazel (*Hamamelis virginiana*), can interfere with your absorption of ephedrine, as can the tannins in tea. Take them two hours apart from this drug.
Bear in Mind:	The side effects of ephedrine, such as nervousness, restlessness, insomnia, and dizziness, may be worsened by caffeine's stimulant effect. Coffee, tea, and cola drinks naturally contain caffeine; it is also added to many soft drinks and "energy-boosting" products. Avoid these when taking ephedrine.

EpiPen, Primatene Mist, others

EPINEPHRINE

Type of Drug:	Bronchodilator
Description:	Epinephrine is the synthetic form of adrenaline. As a nonprescription drug, epinephrine is sold as a mist to be inhaled into the lungs to treat asthma symptoms. If you have asthma, discuss epinephrine with your doctor before you try it. As a prescription drug, epinephrine is sold as EpiPen, an auto injector used for treating anaphylactic shock caused by very severe allergic reactions, such as those caused by bee stings.
Don't Mix With:	Caffeine-containing herbs. The stimulant effect of caffeine can make the side effects of epinephrine, such as nervousness, restlessness, insomnia, and dizziness, worse. Avoid caffeine-containing herbs, including guaraná (*Paullinia cupana*), kola nut (*Cola spp.*), and maté (*Ilex paraguariensis*). Ephedra (*Ephedra spp.*, also known as ma huang). The drug ephedrine, which is very similar to epinephrine, was originally isolated from ephedra. Taking ephedra with any product containing epinephrine could increase the side effects of the drug, including nervousness, insomnia, dizziness, high blood pressure, and heart arrhythmias.
Bear in Mind:	Frequent use of epinephrine mist may lower your levels of vitamin C, potassium, and magnesium. Consider taking supplements (daily multivitamin with minerals). The side effects of epinephrine, such as nervousness, restlessness, insomnia, and dizziness, may be worsened by caffeine's stimulant effect. Coffee, tea, and cola drinks naturally contain caffeine; it is also added to many soft drinks and "energy-boosting" products. Avoid these if taking epinephrine.

ERYTHROMYCIN

Type of Drug:	Macrolide antibiotic

Description:

Erythromycin is used to treat a wide range of bacterial infections and is often prescribed for acne and skin infections. This drug has numerous interactions with other prescription drugs. Be certain to tell your doctor about any other prescription and nonprescription drugs and dietary supplements you take.

If you take any statin drug such as lovastatin (see page 103) or atorvastatin (see page 24), do not take erythromycin. The combination could cause a potentially fatal muscle disease.

Don't Mix With:

Digitalis (*Digitalis spp.*, also known as foxglove). Erythromycin can raise your blood level of both the dangerous herb digitalis and digoxin, a drug with similar effects. Do not mix digitalis and erythromycin.

Bear in Mind:

Erythromycin interferes with your absorption of folic acid, vitamin B6, and vitamin B12, as well as calcium and magnesium. To prevent deficiencies, take a daily multivitamin/mineral supplement at least two hours apart from when you take erythromycin.

Erythromycin kills not only the harmful bacteria that cause illness but also the good bacteria that are normally found in your intestines; this can cause diarrhea. Consider taking probiotic supplements (at least 1.5 billion live organisms daily, including a mixture of *Lactobacillus acidophilus, Bifidobacterium bifidum* and *Saccharomyces boulardii*).

Bromelain, an enzyme found in pineapples, increases your absorption of erythromycin. This may be helpful for people with severe infections or infections that don't respond to erythromycin. Discuss bromelain with your doctor before you try it.

Alora, CombiPatch, Estrace, Estraderm, FemPatch, Vivelle, others

ESTRADIOL

Type of Drug:	Estrogen hormone replacement
Description:	Estradiol is prescribed to replace estrogen in menopausal women. It is used to treat menopause symptoms, such as hot flashes and vaginal dryness, and to help prevent osteoporosis. It is also used to treat some forms of breast cancer and prostate cancer.
Don't Mix With:	Black cohosh (*Cimicifuga racemosa*). Black cohosh contains phytoestrogens, plant hormones similar to human estrogen. Combining it with estradiol could raise your estrogen level too high. Chaste tree (*Vitex agnus-castus*). Chaste tree affects your levels of the hormone prolactin, which in turn can affect estrogen and how your body uses estradiol. Other estrogenic herbs. The herbs dong quai (*Angelica sisis*) and red clover (*Trifolium pratense*) may have estrogen-like effects. Laboratory studies have shown that the herbs licorice (*Glycyrrhiza glabra*), thyme (*Thymus spp.*), turmeric (*Curcuma longa*), hops (*Humulus lupulus*), and vervain (*Verbena spp.*) may also modulate estrogen activity. Discuss the use of these herbs with your medical practitioner before using them if you take estradiol.
Bear in Mind:	Estradiol may block your absorption of folic acid (folate). Consider taking supplements (400 mcg daily). Estradiol may decrease your level of vitamin C, magnesium, and zinc. Consider taking a daily multivitamin with minerals. Studies have shown that soy isoflavones (estrogen-like substances) can help to relieve menopause symptoms. Ipriflavone, a type of soy isoflavone, can help prevent osporosis. Combining soy isoflavones with estradiol could raise your estrogen level too high. If you want to use soy isoflavones in combination with or instead of estradiol, discuss the decision with your doctor first.

Lodine, Lodine XL

ETODOLAC

Type of Drug:	Nonsteroidal anti-inflammatory drug (NSAID)
Description:	Etodolac is an NSAID used to treat arthritis, bursitis, tendinitis, and mild to moderate pain.
Don't Mix With:	No known herbal interactions.
Do Take With:	Deglycyrrhizinated licorice (DGL derived from *Glycyrrhiza glabra*). The soothing and anti-inflammatory properties of DGL can help prevent stomach irritation often caused by etodolac. Consider taking supplements (400 mg 2 to 4 times daily).
Bear in Mind:	Etodolac may cause sodium and water retention. Discuss salt restrictions with your doctor. Etodolac may cause drowsiness, dizziness, or blurred vision. Alcohol can make these side effects worse – don't use it if you take this drug.

Pepcid, Pepcid AC

FAMOTIDINE

Type of Drug:	H2 blocker antacid
Description:	Famotidine sharply reduces your production of stomach acid. In prescription form (Pepcid), it is used to treat ulcers, heartburn, and gastroesophageal reflux disease (GERD). In nonprescription form (Pepcid AC), it is used for mild heartburn.
Don't Mix With:	No known herbal interactions.
Do Take With:	Deglycyrrhizinated licorice (DGL, derived from *Glycyrrhiza glabra*). DGL can speed ulcer healing as it stimulates the production of mucus that protects the stomach lining and also has an antiinflammatory effect. Consider taking supplements (250 mg two to four times daily).
Bear in Mind:	Famotidine and other H2 blockers reduce your absorption of some vitamins and minerals, including folic acid (folate), vitamin B12 (cobalamin), zinc, and iron. If you use these drugs on a regular basis, consider taking supplements (400 mcg daily of folic acid, 500 mcg daily of vitamin B12, plus a daily multivitamin supplement with minerals). Take them at least two hours apart from famotidine. Magnesium supplements and calcium-, magnesium-, and magnesium/aluminum-based antacids may block your absorption of famotidine. Take them at least two hours apart from famotidine.

Prozac

FLUOXETINE

Type of Drug:	Selective serotonin reuptake inhibitor (SSRI)
Description:	Fluoxetine is used to treat depression, obsessive-compulsive disorder, bulimia, anorexia, social phobias, and a number of other disorders. SSRI drugs affect the way your body uses the neurotransmitter serotonin.
Don't Mix With:	Sedative herbs. When combined with fluoxetine, these herbs may cause excessive drowsiness. Avoid sedative herbs such as chamomile (*Matricaria recutita*), catnip (*Nepeta cataria*), kava kava (*Piper methysticum*), passion-flower (*Passiflora incarnata*), St. John's wort (*Hypericum perforatum*), and valerian (*Valeriana officinalis*). St. John's wort (*Hypericum perforatum*). Although there have been no reports of dangerous interactions, it is possible that combining this herb with fluoxetine could raise your serotonin levels too high. This may cause a serious condition called serotonin syndrome. If you wish to take St. John's wort instead of fluoxetine, discuss it with your doctor.
Do Take With:	Ginkgo (*Ginkgo biloba*). Sexual dysfunction in both men and women is a fairly common side effect of fluoxetine. Ginkgo may be helpful in lessening this problem. Consider taking supplements (60 mg *Ginkgo biloba* extract standardized to 24% ginkgo flavone glycosides three times daily).
Bear in Mind:	Don't use the dietary supplements 5-HTP, tryptophan, or SAMe if you take fluoxetine. Both the supplements and the drug increase serotonin levels; it may rise too high, A study in 1995 showed fluoxetine lowers levels of the hormone melatonin. Discuss this with your doctor and consider taking supplements (1 to 3 mg daily). Fluoxetine doesn't work well if your folic acid level is low. Consider taking supplements (400 mcg daily).

Lescol

FLUVASTATIN

Type of Drug:	Statin cholesterol-lowering agent
Description:	Fluvastatin is prescribed to lower high cholesterol, slow or prevent hardening of the arteries, and reduce the risk of heart attack and stroke.
Don't Mix With:	No known herbal interactions.
Do Take With:	Milk thistle (*Silybum marianum*). Although there are no studies of statin drugs to date, silymarin, the active compound in the herb milk thistle, may protect against the liver damage that can occur as a side effect of this type of drug. Consider taking supplements (150 mg three to four times daily).
Bear in Mind:	Lovastatin, a drug similar to fluvastatin, interacts adversely with grapefruit juice. Don't take fluvastatin with grapefruit juice. High doses of niacin (2 to 3 grams daily) can also lower cholesterol. Combining high-dose niacin with some statin drugs, however, can lead to a serious muscle disorder. There are no studies of niacin and fluvastatin, but until more is known, avoid high-dose niacin. The amount of niacin in a daily multivitamin or B vitamin supplement is not enough to cause problems. Red yeast rice, sold as Cholestin, works in a way similar to the statin drugs. Do not use red yeast rice with fluvastatin. According to one study, statin drugs can gradually raise vitamin A levels. Until more is known, don't take vitamin A supplements. The vitamin A contained in a daily multivitamin is not enough to cause problems. Several studies show that taking statin drugs can significantly lower your level of coenzyme Q10 (CoQ10 or ubiquinone), a substance needed for energy production in your cells. Consider taking supplements (100 mg daily).

Luvox

FLUVOXAMINE

Type of Drug:	Selective serotonin reuptake inhibitor (SSRI)
Description:	Fluvoxamine is used to treat obsessive-compulsive disorder and depression. SSRI drugs such as fluvoxamine affect the way your body uses the neurotransmitter serotonin.
Don't Mix With:	Sedative herbs. When combined with fluvoxamine, these herbs may cause excessive drowsiness. Avoid sedative herbs such as chamomile (*Matricaria recutita*), catnip (*Nepeta cataria*), kava kava (*Piper methysticum*), passionflower (Passiflora incarnata), St. John's wort (*Hypericum perforatum*), and valerian (*Valeriana officinalis*). St. John's wort (*Hypericum perforatum*). Although there have been no reports of dangerous interactions, it is possible that combining this herb with fluvoxamine could raise serotonin levels too high. This may cause a serious condition called serotonin syndrome. If you wish to take St. John's wort instead of fluvoxamine, discuss it with your doctor.
Do Take With:	Ginkgo (*Ginkgo*). Sexual dysfunction in both men and women is a fairly common side effect of fluvoxamine. Ginkgo may be helpful in lessening this problem. Consider supplements (60 mg Ginkgo extract standardized to 24% ginkgo flavone glycosides three times daily).
Bear in Mind:	Fluvoxamine can cause drowsiness and dizziness. Alcohol can make these side effects worse. Don't combine the two. Don't use the dietary supplements 5-HTP, tryptophan, or SAMe if you take fluvoxamine. Both the supplements and the drug increase your serotonin level; it may rise too high, causing a serious condition called serotonin syndrome.

Lasix

FUROSEMIDE

Type of Drug:	Loop diuretic

Description: Loop diuretics are used to treat congestive heart failure, high blood pressure, and other conditions such as edema. Furosemide is a powerful diuretic (a drug that removes water from the body) that also depletes your levels of potassium and magnesium. Discuss supplements and your diet with your doctor.

Don't Mix With:

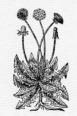

Digitalis (*Digitalis spp.*, also known as foxglove). This dangerous herb is very similar to the heart drug digoxin (see page 61), which can cause dangerous side effects when taken in combination with furosemide. Digitalis can cause the same problem, and should not be combined with furosemide.

Licorice (*Glycyrrhiza glabra*). The potassium-depleting effect of furosemide is worsened by licorice. This effect does not occur with deglycyrrhizinated licorice (DGL) or with artificial licorice flavoring.

Herbal diuretics. Avoid herbal diuretics as their effects, added to that of furosemide, may be dangerous. Herbal diuretics include bilberry leaf (*Vaccinium myrtillus*), buchu (*Barosma betulina*), burdock (*Arctium lappa*), couch grass (*Agropyron repens*), damiana (*Turnera diffusa*), dandelion (*Taraxacum officinale*), fennel seed (*Foeniculum vulgare*), goldenrod (*Solidago virgaurea*), horsetail (*Equisetum arvense*), kava kava (*Piper methysticum*), kola nut (*Cola spp.*), marshmallow (*Althaea officinalis*), maté (*Ilex paraguariensis*), parsley (*Petroselinum spp.*), sarsaparilla (*Smilax spp.*), saw palmetto (*Serenoa repens*), uva ursi (*Arctostaphylos uva ursi*), vervain (*Verbena spp.*), and yarrow (*Achillea millefolium*). Any other nonprescription diuretics should also be avoided.

Lopid, Apo-Gemfibrozil Canada, Novo-Gemfibrozil Canada

GEMFIBROZIL

Type of Drug:	Cholesterol-lowering agent
Description:	Gemfibrozil is prescribed for people with very high triglycerides (a type of blood fat), high LDL cholesterol, and low HDL cholesterol. In general, it is used only when other treatments have failed.
Don't Mix With:	No known herbal interactions.
Bear in Mind:	Red yeast rice. This dietary supplement, sold as Cholestin, works in a way similar to statin drugs, such as lovastatin (see page 103). Combining the statin drugs with gemfibrozil can lead to a potentially fatal muscle disease. Do not combine red yeast rice with gemfibrozil because the same interaction may occur.
	Gemfibrozil may cause dizziness or blurred vision. Alcohol makes these side effects worse. Don't use it in conjunction with this drug.

Garamycin, Genoptic, Ocu-Mycin, others

GENTAMICIN, GENTAMICIN SULFATE

Type of Drug:	Aminoglycoside antibiotic
Description:	Gentamicin is a powerful antibiotic that is given intravenously or by injection (Garamycin) to treat bacterial infections. It is also used in eyedrops to treat eye infections (Genoptic, Ocu-Mycin, others).
Don't Mix With:	No known herbal interactions.
Bear in Mind:	Intravenous or injected gentamicin (but not in eyedrops) kills not only the harmful bacteria that cause illness but also the good bacteria that are normally found in your intestines; this can cause diarrhea. Consider probiotic supplements (at least 1.5 billion live organisms daily, including a mixture of *Lactobacillus acidophilus, Bifidobacterium bifidum,* and *Saccharomyces boulardii*).

Glucotrol, Glucotrol XL

GLIPIZIDE

Type of Drug:	Sulfonylurea antidiabetes drug
Description:	Glipizide is prescribed to lower blood sugar in people with non-insulin-dependent (Type II or adult-onset) diabetes.
Don't Mix With:	No known herbal interactions.
Do Take With: 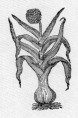	Note: You may be able to reduce the amount of glipizide you need by taking one of the following herbs, or chromium picolinate (see Bear in Mind section). In order to make sure that you are receiving the right amount of medication, it is extremely important for you to discuss your use and dosage of these herbs or this supplement with your doctor before you try them. Fenugreek (*Trigonella foenum-graecum*). In very large doses (25 or more grams daily) fenugreek seeds can help lower blood sugar levels in diabetics. Discuss fenugreek with your doctor before you try it; your glipizide dose may have to be adjusted. Gurmar (*Gymnema sylvestre*). This herb from India may help lower blood sugar levels in diabetics. Consider taking supplements (100 mg three times daily). Discuss Gurmar with your doctor before you try it; your glipizide dose may have to be adjusted. Other herbs. Bitter melon (*Momordica charantia*), burdock (*Arctium lappa*), dandelion (*Taraxacum officinale*), garlic (*Allium sativum*), and ginseng (*Panax ginseng*) are among the herbs that are traditionally recommended for lowering blood sugar in diabetics. Use these herbs with caution and discuss them with your doctor first. Your glipizide dose may have to be adjusted.
Bear in Mind:	The mineral chromium can be helpful for lowering blood sugar in diabetics. Consider taking supplements in the form of chromium picolinate (500 to 1,000 mcg daily). Discuss chromium picolinate with your doctor before you try it; your glipizide dose may have to be adjusted.

DiaBeta, Glynase Pres Tab, Micronase

GLYBURIDE

Type of Drug:	Sulfonylurea antidiabetes drug
Description:	Glyburide is prescribed to lower blood sugar in people with non-insulin-dependent (Type II or adult-onset) diabetes.
Don't Mix With:	No known herbal interactions.
Do Take With:	Note: You may be able to reduce the amount of glyburide you need by taking one of the following herbs, or chromium picolinate (see Bear in Mind section). In order to make sure that you are receiving the right amount of medication, it is extremely important for you to discuss your use and dosage of these herbs or this supplement with your doctor before you try them.

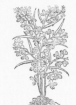

	Fenugreek (*Trigonella foenum-graecum*). In very large doses (25 or more grams daily) fenugreek seeds can help lower blood sugar levels in diabetics. Discuss fenugreek with your doctor before you try it; your glyburide dose may have to be adjusted.
	Gurmar (*Gymnema sylvestre*). This herb from India may help lower blood sugar levels in diabetics. Discuss Gurmar with your doctor before you try it; your glyburide dose may have to be adjusted. Consider taking supplements (100 mg three times daily).
	Other herbs. Bitter melon (*Momordica charantia*), burdock (*Arctium lappa*), dandelion (*Taraxacum officinale*), garlic (*Allium sativum*), and ginseng (*Panax ginseng*) are among the herbs that are traditionally recommended for lowering blood sugar in diabetics. Use these herbs with caution and discuss them with your doctor first. Your glyburide dose may have to be adjusted.
Bear in Mind:	The mineral chromium can be helpful for lowering blood sugar in diabetics. Consider taking supplements in the form of chromium picolinate (500 to 1,000 mcg daily). Discuss this with your doctor first; the glyburide dose may have to be adjusted.

Haldol

HALOPERIDOL

Type of Drug:	Antipsychotic
Description:	Haloperidol is prescribed to treat psychotic disorders, schizophrenia, Tourette's syndrome, and acute psychiatric conditions.
Don't Mix With: 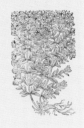	Caffeine-containing herbs. Research suggests that caffeine can reduce your absorption of haloperidol. Do not use the caffeine-containing herbs guaraná (*Paullinia cupana*), kola nut (*Cola spp.*), and maté (*Ilex paraguariensis*) within two hours of taking this drug. Sedative herbs. When combined with haloperidol, sedative herbs may cause excessive drowsiness. Avoid sedative herbs such as chamomile (*Matricaria recutita*), catnip (*Nepeta cataria*), kava kava (*Piper methysticum*), passionflower (*Passiflora incarnata*), St. John's wort (*Hypericum perforatum*), valerian (*Valeriana officinalis*), and others, as well as sedative dietary supplements such as 5-HTP, tryptophan, and SAMe.
Bear in Mind:	Haloperidol can cause drowsiness. Alcohol can make this side effect worse. Don't use it in conjunction with this drug. Caffeine may reduce the absorption of haloperidol. Coffee, tea, chocolate, and cola drinks naturally contain caffeine; it is also added to many soft drinks and "energy-boosting" products. Avoid these drinks and products for two hours before and after taking haloperidol.

This drug is sold as a generic only.

HEPARIN

Type of Drug:	Anticoagulant
Description:	Heparin is a very powerful blood-thinning drug that is given by injection to prevent and treat blood clots. Be sure to tell your medical practitioner about any prescription or nonprescription drugs, and herbs or supplements you are taking.
Don't Mix With:	Blood-thinning herbs. A number of herbs have known or possible anticoagulant action and may cause an increased risk of bleeding when used with heparin. Avoid dan shen (*Salvia miltiorrhiza*), devil's claw (*Harpagophytum procumbens*), garlic (*Allium sativum*), ginger (*Zingiber officinale*), ginkgo (*Ginkgo biloba*), ginseng (*Panax ginseng*), and sweet woodruff (*Galium odoratum*). Foods containing garlic and ginger in moderate amounts are unlikely to cause any problems. In addition, the herbs dong quai (*Angelica sinensis*), fenugreek (*Trigonella foenum-graecum*), horse chestnut (*Aesculus hippocastanum*), and red clover (*Trifolium pratense*) contain small amounts of chemicals similar to warfarin, another powerful blood-thinning drug (see page 156), and should be avoided when taking heparin.
Bear in Mind:	High doses of vitamin C (more than 3,000 mg daily) might reduce the blood-thinning effect of heparin. High doses of vitamin E may cause an increased risk of bleeding when used with heparin. In addition, dietary supplements such as phosphatidyl serine and fish oil may interact adversely with heparin. In general, avoid any dietary supplements when taking heparin unless you have discussed them with your medical practitioner.

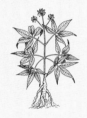

Apresoline
HYDRALAZINE

Type of Drug:	Antihypertensive
Description:	Hydralazine is usually prescribed to lower high blood pressure. It is sometimes prescribed to treat congestive heart failure. This drug can make some heart problems worse and could cause angina or a heart attack. Be certain to tell your doctor if you have ever had any heart trouble.
Don't Mix With:	Blood vessel relaxing herbs. *Coleus forskohlii,* garlic (*Allium sativum*), ginkgo (*Ginkgo biloba*), and hawthorn (*Crataegus monogyna*) relax your blood vessels and are sometimes used to treat high blood pressure. Although there have been no studies, it's possible that combining these herbs with hydralazine could make your blood pressure drop too low.
Bear in Mind:	Hydralazine works by opening up your blood vessels. Alcohol has a similar effect. Don't combine alcohol with this drug because your blood pressure may drop too low. Hydralazine can make you eliminate extra Vitamin B6 (pyridoxine), which could cause a deficiency. Discuss this with your doctor and consider taking supplements (50 mg daily).

Cortef, Hydrocortone

HYDROCORTISONE

Type of Drug:	Corticosteroid
Description:	Corticosteroids such as hydrocortisone are synthetic hormones used to treat a wide variety of severe disorders, particularly those that involve inflammation, including arthritis, psoriasis, allergies, asthma, and inflammatory bowel disease. They also treat autoimmune diseases such as lupus erythematosus and transplant rejection. Hydrocortisone in small amounts is used in many nonprescription creams to relieve itching from poison ivy, insect bites, mild psoriasis, and other minor skin irritations. The amount of hydrocortisone in these creams is not enough to cause interactions in most people.
Don't Mix With:	Digitalis (*Digitalis spp.*, also known as foxglove). This dangerous herb is very similar to the heart drug digoxin (see page 61), which may worsen the side effects of hydrocortisone. Digitalis may cause the same problem. Ephedra (*Ephedra spp.*, also known as ma huang). The herb ephedra naturally contains ephedrine, which can reduce the effectiveness of corticosteroids. Do not use it when taking hydrocortisone. Similarly, avoid the drugs ephedrine (see page 71) and pseudoephedrine (see page 136), found in many nonprescription cold and allergy remedies.
Bear in Mind:	Corticosteroids can cause the retention of sodium, which is found in salt. Discuss salt restrictions with your doctor. Long-term use of corticosteroids may cause osteoporosis. Consider taking supplements (1,000 mg calcium daily, 400 IU vitamin D daily). Corticosteroids may also reduce your levels of vitamin B6 (pyridoxine) and magnesium. Consider taking supplements (50 mg pyridoxine daily and 300-400 mg magnesium daily). Because this drug reduces your level of chromium, long-term use of corticosteroids may contribute to the development of diabetes. Consider taking supplements (200 mcg chromium picolinate daily).

Advil, Arthritis Foundation, Midol, Motrin, Nuprin, others

IBUPROFEN

Type of Drug:	Nonsteroidal antiinflammatory drug (NSAID)
Description:	Ibuprofen is an NSAID used to treat arthritis, headaches, menstrual discomfort, and mild to moderate pain. It is also used to treat fever and swelling. Ibuprofen is sold as both a prescription drug (Motrin) and nonprescription drug (Advil, Arthritis Foundation, Midol, Nuprin, others).
Don't Mix With:	No known herbal interactions.
Do Take With:	Deglycyrrhizinated licorice (DGL, derived from *Glycyrrhiza glabra*). DGL stimulates the production of mucus that protects the stomach lining and also has an antiinflammatory effect. It may help prevent the stomach irritation often caused by ibuprofen. Consider taking supplements (400 mg two to four times daily).
Bear In Mind:	Ibuprofen can irritate your stomach. Alcohol can make this effect worse. Don't combine alcohol with this drug. Take ibuprofen with food to reduce the risk of stomach irritation.

Tofranil, Tofranil-PM

IMIPRAMINE

Type of Drug:	Tricyclic antidepressant
Description:	Imipramine is used to treat depression. Like other tricyclic antidepressants, it works by affecting the way chemicals called neurotransmitters, including serotonin and norepinephrine, move in and out of your nerve endings.
Don't Mix With:	Ephedra (*Ephedra spp.*, also known as ma huang). Taking ephedra with any tricyclic antidepressant increases your risk of serious high blood pressure and heart arrhythmias. Similarly, avoid the related drugs ephedrine and pseudoephedrine, which are found in many nonprescription cold and allergy remedies. Sedative herbs. Sedative herbs may cause excessive drowsiness when combined with imipramine. Avoid sedative herbs such as chamomile (*Matricaria recutita*), catnip (*Nepeta cataria*), kava kava (*Piper methysticum*), passionflower (*Passiflora incarnata*), St. John's wort (*Hypericum perforatum*), valerian (*Valeriana officinalis*), and others, as well as sedative dietary supplements such as 5-HTP, tryptophan, and SAMe. St. John's wort (*Hypericum perforatum*). Research suggests that this herb and imipramine work in similar ways. Until more is known, don't take imipramine in conjunction with St. John's wort. Yohimbe. (*Pausinystalia yohimbe*) This dangerous herb is said to improve male sexual function. Don't use this herb when taking imipramine; the combination may cause a dangerous rise in blood pressure.
Bear in Mind:	Heart problems can be a side effect of tricyclic antidepressants, possibly because these drugs lower your production of coenzyme Q10 (CoQ10 or ubiquinone). Consider taking supplements (20 to 50 mg daily).

Crixivan

INDINAVIR

Type of Drug:	Antiviral
Description:	Indinavir is used in combination with the antiviral drug AZT (see page 27) as part of a "cocktail" of drugs to treat HIV infection and AIDS. Indinavir has a number of serious side effects, including increased cholesterol and blood glucose levels. Indinavir can interact adversely with a number of drugs, including drugs to control cholesterol and triglycerides. Be certain to tell you doctor about any other prescription and nonprescription drugs and dietary supplements you take.
Don't Mix With:	St. John's wort (*Hypericum perforatum*). Your absorption of protease inhibitors is seriously reduced by this herb. Do not use it if you are taking indinavir.
Do Take With:	Milk thistle (*Silybum marianum*). Silymarin, the active compound in the herb milk thistle, may help protect your liver against damage from indinavir. Discuss this with your medical practitioner and consider taking supplements (200 mg daily).
Bear in Mind:	Indinavir works best if you take it on an empty stomach. Fatty foods block your absorption of the drug. To avoid the risk of kidney stones, drink plenty of liquids (at least 64 ounces a day).

Indochron E-R, Indocin, Indocin SR

INDOMETHACIN

Type of Drug:	Nonsteroidal antiinflammatory drug (NSAID)
Description:	Indomethacin is a prescription NSAID used to treat arthritis, tendinitis, bursitis, menstrual discomfort, and migraine. It can interact adversely with many drugs frequently prescribed for high blood pressure and heart problems. Be certain to tell your doctor about all prescription and nonprescription drugs and dietary supplements you take.
Don't Mix With:	No known herbal interactions.
Do Take With:	Deglycyrrhizinated licorice (DGL, derived from *Glycyrrhiza glabra*). DGL stimulates the production of mucus that protects the stomach lining and also has an antiinflammatory effect. It may help prevent the stomach irritation often caused by indomethacin. Consider taking supplements (400 mg two to four times daily).
Bear In Mind:	Indomethacin can irritate your stomach. Alcohol can make this effect worse. Don't combine alcohol with this drug. Take indomethacin with food to reduce the risk of stomach irritation. Indomethacin may reduce your absorption of vitamins and minerals such as vitamin C and calcium. Consider taking a daily multivitamin supplement with minerals at least two hours apart from the drug.

Fluogen, Flu-Shield, Fluvirin, Fluzone

INFLUENZA VACCINE

Type of Drug:	Influenza vaccine
Description:	Influenza vaccines are administered as a protective measure against catching the flu; they may also keep the flu from being as severe if you do catch it. The vaccines are modified annually to protect against the flu strains researchers believe are most likely to occur that season.
Don't Mix With:	No known herbal interactions.
Do Take With:	Ginseng (*Panax ginseng*). A well-conducted study in 1996 showed that ginseng may help the flu vaccine work better by increasing antibody production and decreasing the frequency of colds and flus. The dose used in the study was 100 mg taken twice daily for four weeks before vaccination and eight weeks afterward.

Humalog, Humulin, Iletin, Novolin, Velosulin, others

INSULIN

Type of Drug:	Antidiabetic
Description:	Insulin drugs are very similar to the hormone insulin produced by your pancreas. They are used by people with insulin-dependent (juvenile or type 1 diabetes) diabetes to replace the insulin their pancreas doesn't make. These drugs are also used by some people with non-insulin-dependent (adult-onset or type 2) diabetes. Insulin must be injected. Because many drugs interact with insulin, be certain to tell your doctor about any prescription and nonprescription and dietary supplements you take.
Don't Mix With:	No known herbal interactions.
Do Take With:	Note: You may be able to reduce the amount of insulin you need by taking one of the following herbs. In order to make sure that you are receiving the right amount of medication, it is extremely important for you to discuss your use and dosage of these herbs or this supplement with your doctor before you try them. Fenugreek (*Trigonella foenum-graecum*). In very large doses (25 or more grams daily) fenugreek seeds can help lower blood sugar levels in diabetics. Discuss fenugreek with your doctor before you try it; your insulin dose may have to be adjusted. Gurmar (*Gymnema sylvestre*). This herb from India may help lower blood sugar levels in diabetics. Consider taking supplements (100 mg three times daily). Discuss gurmar with your doctor before you try it; your insulin dose may have to be adjusted. Other herbs: Bitter melon (*Momordica charantia*), burdock (*Arctium lappa*), dandelion (*Taraxacum officinale*), garlic (*Allium sativum*), and ginseng (*Panax ginseng*) are among the herbs that are traditionally recommended for lowering blood sugar in diabetics. Use these herbs with caution and discuss them with your doctor first. The insulin dose may have to be adjusted.

Actimmune, Alferon N, Avonex, Betaseron, Rebif, others

INTERFERON

Type of Drug:	Antiviral
Description:	Interferon is an antiviral drug prescribed for hepatitis C and other viral infections. It is also used to treat multiple sclerosis, some kinds of cancer, and other diseases. Because interferon can cause liver damage and other problems, you will need to be carefully monitored by your medical practitioner.
Don't Mix With:	Bupleurum (*Bupleurum spp.*). Combining bupleurum in any form with interferon can lead to a dangerous form of lung disease. Never mix the two. This herb, also known as hare's ear (chai hu) or thorewax root, is sometimes recommended by herbalists for a wide variety of ailments. It is found in some Japanese herbal combination formulas for treating liver disease, including the products known as sho-saiko-to (TJ-9) and xino-chai-hu-tang.
Bear in Mind:	Preliminary research indicates that it is possible that the dietary supplement n-acetyl-cysteine (NAC) may enhance the effectiveness of interferon. Discuss this with your medical practitioner and consider taking supplements (600 mg three times daily).

INH, Laniazid, Nydrazid, Rifamate, Rimactane

ISONIAZID

Type of Drug:	Antitubercular
Description:	Isoniazid, either by itself (INH, Laniazid) or in combination with rifampin (Rifamate, Rimactane) is an antibiotic prescribed to treat tuberculosis.
Don't Mix With:	St. John's wort (*Hypericum perforatum*). Isoniazid has some effects similar to monoamine oxidase inhibitor (MAOI) drugs. St. John's wort may work in a way similar to these drugs. Until more is known, do not mix St. John's wort with isoniazid. The combination could worsen isoniazid's side effects, including flu-like symptoms, nausea, dizziness, drowsiness, and headache.
Bear in Mind:	Combining alcohol with isoniazid can cause a number of unpleasant side effects, including headache and nausea.
	Isoniazid has some effects similar to monoamine oxidase inhibitor (MAOI) drugs such as phenelzine (see page 126). Like MAOI drugs, isoniazid may interact adversely with foods containing the amino acid tyramine, such as alcohol, cheese and other dairy foods, fermented foods such as sauerkraut and pickles, bologna, salami, pepperoni, liver, pickled herring, caffeine, and chocolate. Symptoms include diarrhea, vasodilation (flushing), and dangerous changes in your blood pressure, among others. Discuss food restrictions with your doctor and follow them carefully.
	Combining isoniazid with supplements of the amino acid tryptophan, sold as 5-HTP and often used as a natural sedative, may cause excessive drowsiness.
	Isoniazid can interfere with the action of vitamin B6 (pyridoxine) and the absorption of other vitamins and minerals. Consider taking a daily multivitamin and mineral supplement containing 50 mg of vitamin B6 at least two hours apart from the drug.

Dilatrate-SR, Imdur, ISMO, Isordil, Monoket, Sorbitrate

ISOSORBIDE DINITRATE

Type of Drug:	Antianginal
Description:	Isosorbide is prescribed to relieve the heart or chest pain of angina and to treat congestive heart failure and some other heart problems. This drug is sometimes used in sublingual (under the tongue) tablets to provide immediate relief from angina pain.
Don't Mix With:	No known herbal interactions.
Bear in Mind:	One study in 1989 suggested that the dietary supplement n-acetyl-cysteine (NAC) may help isosorbide work better. Discuss NAC supplements with your doctor before you try them.

Accutane

ISOTRETINOIN

Type of Drug:	Antiacne
Description:	Isotretinoin is a modified form of vitamin A. It is prescribed to treat severe acne.
Don't Mix With:	No known herbal interactions.
Bear in Mind:	Isotretinoin can cause birth defects. Women of childbearing age should not take this drug unless they are certain they are not pregnant and are using effective contraception.
	About 25 percent of people who take isotretinoin develop high triglycerides (a type of blood fat). Discuss this possibility with your doctor.
	Large amounts of vitamin A, in addition to isotretinoin, lead to the risk of vitamin A toxicity. Do not take vitamin A supplements or eat liver or foods made with liver, which are very high in vitamin A, while you are taking this drug. Before taking a multivitamin, or any supplement containing vitamin A, discuss it with your doctor.

Prevacid
LANSOPRAZOLE

Type of Drug:	Proton pump inhibitor antacid
Description:	Lansoprazole "turns off" your production of stomach acid. It is used to treat ulcers, severe heartburn, and gastroesophageal reflux disease (GERD).
Don't Mix With:	No known herbal interactions.
Do Take With:	Deglycyrrhizinated licorice (DGL, derived from *Glycyrrhiza glabra*). DGL can speed ulcer healing as it stimulates the production of mucus that protects the stomach lining and also has an antiinflammatory effect. Consider taking supplements (250 mg two to four times daily).
Bear in Mind:	Lansoprazole may block your absorption of certain vitamins and minerals, particularly folic acid (folate), vitamin B12 (cobalamin), and iron. If you use lansoprazole or other proton pump inhibitors on a regular basis, take a multivitamin supplement with minerals at least two hours apart from taking the drug, and additional folic acid (400 mcg daily) and vitamin B12 (500 mcg daily).

Eltroxin, Levo-T, Levothroid, Levoxine, Levoxyl, Synthroid

LEVOTHYROXINE

Type of Drug:	Synthetic thyroid hormone replacement
Description:	Levothyroxine is a synthetic hormone prescribed for hypothyroidism (underactive thyroid gland). Levothyroxine may interact adversely with some drugs. Be certain to tell your doctor about any prescription and nonprescription drugs and dietary supplements you take.
Don't Mix With:	Bugleweed (*Lycopus spp.*). This herb may interfere with the action of thyroid hormones, including levothyroxine. Lemon balm (*Melissa officinalis*). This herb may interfere with the action of thyroid hormones, including levothyroxine.
Bear in Mind:	While iron supplements may help improve thyroid function, they can also reduce your absorption of levothyroxine. Discuss iron supplements with your doctor. If you decide to take supplements, it is very important to take them at least two hours apart from levothyroxine. Soy foods may block your absorption of levothyroxine. Do not eat these foods within two hours of taking the drug. Take levothyroxine at the same time every day, preferably before breakfast. Wait at least 30 to 60 minutes before taking any other supplements.

Eskalith, Lithobid, Lithonate, Lithotabs

LITHIUM

Type of Drug:	Antipsychotic, antimanic
Description:	Lithium is prescribed for bipolar disorder (manic depression) and severe depression.

Don't Mix With:

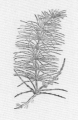

Caffeine-containing herbs. In combination with lithium, caffeine may raise blood levels of the drug and may exacerbate hand tremors caused by it. Avoid caffeine-containing herbs, including guaraná (*Paullinia cupana*), kola nut (*Cola nitida*), and maté (*Ilex paraguariensis*).

Diuretic herbs. Combining lithium and diuretic herbs increases the risk of side effects such as electrolyte disturbances and frequent urination. Avoid diuretic herbs including bilberry leaf (*Vaccinium myrtillus*), buchu (*Barosma betulina*), burdock (*Arctium lappa*), couch grass (*Agropyron repens*), damiana (*Turnera diffusa*), dandelion (*Taraxacum officinale*), fennel seed (*Foeniculum vulgare*), goldenrod (*Solidago virgaurea*), horsetail (*Equisetum arvense*), kava kava (*Piper methysticum*), kola nut (*Cola nitida*), marshmallow (*Althaea officinalis*), maté (Ilex paraguariensis), parsley (*Petroselinum crispum*), sarsaparilla (*Smilax spp.*), saw palmetto (*Serenoa repens*), uva ursi (*Arctostaphylos uva ursi*), vervain (*Verbena officinalis*), and yarrow (*Achillea millefolium*). Any other prescription or nonprescription diuretics should also be avoided,

Bear in Mind:

Caffeine can raise blood levels of lithium, increasing the risk of adverse side effects. Avoid coffee, tea, and cola drinks naturally containing caffeine, as of many soft drinks and "energy-boosting" products. Avoid these if taking lithium.

Some studies show that taking folic acid (folate) supplements (400 mcg daily) can increase the beneficial effects of lithium.

Nonsteroidal anti-inflammatory drugs (NSAIDs), such as aspirin (see page 22), ibuprofen (see page 80), and indomethacin (see page 92), may decrease the excretion rate of lithium, leading to a potentially dangerous increase in levels of the drug. Do not take NSAIDS with lithium.

Claritin, Claritin-D, Claritin Reditabs

LORATADINE

Type of Drug:	Antihistamine
Description:	Loratadine is an antihistamine used to treat the symptoms of seasonal allergies, such as sneezing, runny nose, and itchy eyes. It is also used to treat other allergy symptoms such as itching, rashes, and hives. In some cases, it is used to treat asthma. One preparation containing loratadine, Claritin-D, also contains pseudoephedrine (see page 136).
Don't Mix With:	Henbane (*Hyoscyamus niger*). This herb is toxic and should be used only when prescribed and closely monitored by a qualified practitioner. Although loratadine has few side effects, it can cause headache, dry mouth, and drowsiness. Henbane could make these side effects worse. Sedative herbs. Loratadine causes drowsiness in some people. Combining sedative herbs with loratidine could cause excessive drowsiness. Avoid herbs such as chamomile (*Matricaria recutita*), catnip (*Nepeta cataria*), kava kava (*Piper methysticum*), passionflower (*Passiflora incarnata*), St. John's wort (*Hypericum perforatum*), valerian (*Valeriana officinalis*), and others, as well as sedative dietary supplements such as 5-HTP, tryptophan, and SAMe.
Bear in Mind:	Loratadine is less likely than most other antihistamines to cause drowsiness, but it can have a sedative effect in some people. Alcohol will make the drowsiness worse. Don't use it if taking this drug.

Mevacor

LOVASTATIN

Type of Drug:	Statin cholesterol-lowering agent
Description:	Lovastatin is prescribed to lower high cholesterol, to slow or prevent hardening of the arteries, and to reduce the risk of heart attack and stroke.
Don't Mix With:	No known herbal interactions.
Do Take With:	Milk thistle (*Silybum marianum*). Although there are no studies of statin drugs to date, silymarin, the active compound in the herb milk thistle may protect against the liver damage that can occur as a side effect of this drug. Consider taking supplements (150 mg three to four times daily).
Bear in Mind:	A study in 1998 showed that lovastatin interacts adversely with grapefruit juice and could cause a serious muscle disease. Do not take lovastatin with grapefruit juice. The dietary supplement red yeast rice, sold as Cholestin, works in a way similar to the statin drugs. Do not use red yeast rice when taking lovastatin. According to one study, statin drugs can gradually raise vitamin A levels. Until more is known, don't take vitamin A supplements with lovastatin. Several studies show that taking statin drugs can significantly lower your level of coenzyme Q10 (CoQ10 or ubiquinone), a substance needed for energy production in the cells. Consider taking supplements (100 mg daily). Some research suggests that moderate doses of niacin (500 mg three times daily) can have a supportive effect on lovastatin. Discuss niacin with your doctor before you try it, however, because high doses of niacin interact adversely with some statin drugs.

Glucophage

METFORMIN

Type of Drug:	Biguanide antidiabetes drug
Description:	Metformin is prescribed to lower blood sugar in people with non-insulin-dependent (Type II or adult-onset) diabetes. It is sometimes used in combined with glipizide (see page 83) or glyburide (see page 84).
Don't Mix With:	No known herbal interactions.
Do Take With: 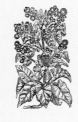	Note: You may be able to reduce the amount of metformin you need by taking one of the following herbs, or chromium picolinate (see Bear in Mind section). In order to make sure that you are receiving the right amount of medication, it is extremely important for you to discuss your use and dosage of these herbs or this supplement with your doctor before you try them.
	Fenugreek (*Trigonella foenum-graecum*). In very large doses (25 or more grams daily) fenugreek seeds can help lower blood sugar levels in diabetics. Discuss fenugreek with your doctor before you try it; your metformin dose may have to be adjusted.
	Gurmar (*Gymnema sylvestre*). This herb from India may help lower blood sugar levels in diabetics. Discuss gurmar with your doctor before you try it; your metformin dose may have to be adjusted. Consider taking supplements (100 mg three times daily).
	Other herbs. Bitter melon (*Momordica charantia*), burdock (*Arctium lappa*), dandelion (*Taraxacum officinale*), garlic (*Allium sativum*), and ginseng (*Panax ginseng*) are among the herbs that are traditionally recommended for lowering blood sugar in diabetics. Use these herbs with caution and discuss them with your doctor first. Your metformin dose may have to be adjusted.
Bear in Mind:	Metformin can lower your levels of folic acid (folate) and vitamin B12. Consider taking supplements (folic acid 400 mcg daily; vitamin B12 500 mcg daily).

Folex, Rheumatrex

METHOTREXATE

Type of Drug:	Antiarthritic, antiinflammatory
Description:	Methotrexate is prescribed to treat severe rheumatoid arthritis, severe psoriasis, and some forms of cancer. It is also sometimes used to treat severe asthma. Methotrexate is a powerful drug that works by blocking your use of the B vitamin folic acid (folate). This drug can have severe, life-threatening side effects. Be certain to discuss the possible side effects with your doctor, as well as any other prescription or nonprescription drugs or supplements you are taking.
Don't Mix With:	Salicylate-containing herbs. The herbs meadowsweet (*Filipendula ulmaria*), white willow bark (*Salix alba*), and wintergreen (*Gaultheria procumbens*) contain salicylate, a chemical similar to aspirin. Taking these herbs with methotrexate could increase its action, leading to possible toxicity. Discuss aspirin and other nonsteroidal anti-inflammatory drugs (NSAIDs) such as ibuprofen (see page 80), ketoprofen, and naproxen (see page 109) with your doctor.
Bear in Mind:	Methotrexate blocks your absorption of folic acid (folate), vitamin B12 (cobalamin), and beta carotene. Discuss supplements with your doctor – do not take supplements of these vitamins on your own. Riboflavin (Vitamin B2) may reduce the effectiveness of methotrexate. Do not take riboflavin supplements if you are taking methotrexate. Don't mix alcohol with methotrexate – liver damage may occur.

Aldomet

METHYLDOPA

Type of Drug:	Antihypertensive
Description:	Methyldopa is prescribed to lower high blood pressure. This drug is usually taken along with another medication to treat high blood pressure, such as a diuretic.

Don't Mix With:

Herbal diuretics. Combining methyldopa and diuretic herbs increases the risk of side effects such as electrolyte disturbances and dehydration. Avoid herbal diuretics including bilberry leaf (*Vaccinium myrtillus*), buchu (*Barosma betulina*), burdock (*Arctium lappa*), couch grass (*Agropyron repens*), damiana (*Turnera diffusa*), dandelion (*Taraxacum officinale*), fennel seed (*Foeniculum vulgare*), goldenrod (*Solidago virgaurea*), horsetail (*Equisetum arvense*), kava kava (*Piper methysticum*), kola nut (*Cola spp.*), marshmallow (*Althaea officinalis*), maté (*Ilex paraguariensis*), parsley (*Petroselinum spp.*), sarsaparilla (*Smilax spp.*), saw palmetto (*Serenoa repens*), uva ursi (*Arctostaphylos uva ursi*), vervain (*Verbena spp.*), and yarrow (*Achillea millefolium*). Any other prescription or nonprescription diuretics should also be avoided, except on medical advice.

Sedative herbs. When combined with methyldopa, sedative herbs may cause excessive drowsiness. Avoid chamomile (*Matricaria recutita*), catnip (*Nepeta cataria*), kava kava (*Piper methysticum*), passionflower (*Passiflora incarnata*), St. John's wort (*Hypericum perforatum*), valerian (*Valeriana officinalis*), and others, as well as sedative dietary supplements such as 5-HTP, tryptophan, and SAMe.

Bear in Mind:

Iron supplements can decrease your absorption of methyldopa. Take iron supplements two hours apart from the drug.

Methyldopa can lower your level of vitamin B12. To avoid a deficiency, consider supplements (500 mcg daily).

A low-salt diet will help methyldopa work better. Discuss your salt intake with your doctor.

Ritalin, Ritalin SR

METHYLPHENIDATE HYDROCHLORIDE

Type of Drug:	Central nervous system stimulant
Description:	Methylphenidate is a stimulant drug similar to amphetamines. It is often prescribed to children to treat attention deficit hyperactivity disorder (ADHD). It is also used for some psychological, social, and learning disorders. Although methylphenidate is a stimulant, when given to children it usually has a mildly sedating effect.
Don't Mix With:	Caffeine-containing herbs. The stimulant effect of caffeine could interact adversely with methylphenidate. Avoid caffeine-containing herbs, including guaraná (*Paullinia cupana*), kola nut (*Cola spp.*), and maté (*Ilex paraguariensis*). Sedative herbs. Although there have been no studies of how natural sedatives interact with methylphenidate, it is possible these herbs could increase the sedative effect of the drug. Until more is known, avoid sedative herbs such as chamomile (*Matricaria recutita*), catnip (*Nepeta cataria*), kava kava (*Piper methysticum*), passionflower (*Passiflora incarnata*), St. John's wort (*Hypericum perforatum*), valerian (*Valeriana officinalis*), and others, as well as sedative dietary supplements such as 5-HTP, tryptophan, and SAMe.
Bear in Mind:	The stimulant effect of caffeine could interact adversely with methylphenidate. Coffee, tea, and cola drinks naturally contain caffeine; it is also added to many soft drinks and "energy-boosting" products. Avoid these products if taking this drug. Methylphenidate can cause drowsiness. This side effect is worsened by alcohol. Avoid alcohol when taking this drug.

Flagyl, Helidac, MetroGel, Protostat, others

METRONIDAZOLE

Type of Drug:	Antibiotic
Description:	Metronidazole is an antibiotic used to treat bacterial, fungal, and parasitic infections, particularly infections of the vagina, bone, brain, and urinary tract. In combination with bismuth subsalicylate (see page 29) and tetracycline (see page 146), metronidazole (Flagyl) is used to treat ulcers caused by Helicobacter pylori infection.
Don't Mix With:	No known herbal interactions.
Do Take With:	Deglycyrrhizinated licorice (DGL, derived from *Glycyrrhiza glabra*). DGL can speed ulcer healing as it stimulates the production of mucus that protects the stomach lining and also has an antiinflammatory effect. Consider taking supplements (400 mg two to four times daily). Milk thistle (*Silybum marianum*). Silymarin, the active compound in the herb milk thistle, may help protect your liver against damage from metronidazole. Consider supplements (200 mg daily).
Bear in Mind:	Metronidazole kills not only the harmful bacteria that cause illness but also the good bacteria that are normally found in your intestines; this can cause diarrhea. Consider taking probiotic supplements (at least 1.5 billion live organisms daily, including a mixture of *Lactobacillus acidophilus, Bifidobacterium bifidum,* and *Saccharomyces boulardii*). Do not drink alcohol while taking metronidazole. Severe side effects, including vasodilation (flushing), headache, and nausea may occur. Vinegar may have a similar effect. Avoid salad dressings, pickles, and other foods containing vinegar.

Aleve, Anaprox, Naprelan, Naprosyn, others

NAPROXEN

Type of Drug:	Nonsteroidal antiinflammatory drug (NSAID)
Description:	Naproxen is used mostly to relieve pain, swelling, and stiffness from arthritis, tendinitis, and bursitis. It's also used to lower fevers, relieve menstrual discomfort, and to treat mild to moderate pain. Naproxen is available in prescription (Anaprox, Naprelan, Naprosyn, others) and nonprescription (Aleve, others) strengths.
Don't Mix With:	No known herbal interactions.
Do Take With:	Deglycyrrhizinated licorice (DGL, derived from *Glycyrrhiza glabra*) stimulates the production of mucus that protects the stomach lining and also has an antiinflammatory effect. It may help prevent the stomach irritation often caused by naproxen. Consider taking supplements (400 mg two to four times daily).
Bear In Mind:	Naproxen can raise the amount of potassium in your body. Avoid potassium supplements or salt substitutes while taking this drug. Discuss your intake of foods high in potassium, such as bananas and orange juice, with your medical practitioner. Naproxen may make you retain sodium and water. Discuss salt restriction with your doctor. Naproxen may cause drowsiness, dizziness, or blurred vision. Alcohol can make these side effects worse – don't use it if taking this drug. Take naproxen with food to avoid stomach irritation.

Serzone

NEFAZODONE

Type of Drug:	Antidepressant
Description:	Nefazodone is prescribed to treat depression.
Don't Mix With: 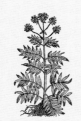	Digitalis (*Digitalis spp.*, also known as foxglove). This dangerous herb is very similar to the heart drug digoxin (see page 61). Nefazodone increases the amount of digoxin in your blood, possibly to dangerous levels, and may have the same effect with digitalis. Do not use this herb if taking nefazodone.
	Sedative herbs. Although there have been no studies, it is possible that nefazodone in combination with natural sedatives could cause excessive drowsiness. Until more is known, avoid sedative herbs such as chamomile (*Matricaria recutita*), catnip (*Nepeta cataria*), kava kava (*Piper methysticum*), passionflower (*Passiflora incarnata*), valerian (*Valeriana officinalis*), and others, as well as sedative dietary supplements such as 5-HTP, tryptophan, and SAMe, when taking nefazodone.
	St. John's wort (*Hypericum perforatum*). St. John's wort and nefazodone may work in similar ways. To avoid increasing the effect of the drug, don't take St. John's wort.
Bear in Mind:	Do not combine nefazodone with alcohol. The combination may cause dangerous drowsiness.

Habitrol, Nicoderm, Nicorette, Nicotrol, ProStep

NICOTINE

Type of Drug:	Smoking cessation product
Description:	Nicotine replacement products are used to help people quit smoking by easing the symptoms of nicotine withdrawal. Nicotine is available as a prescription skin patch (Habitrol), as a nonprescription chewing gum (Nicorette), and as a nonprescription skin patch (Nicoderm, Nicotrol, ProStep).
	Nicotine overdose can be dangerous and even fatal. Follow the directions given by your doctor or the package insert.
Don't Mix With:	Lobelia (*Lobelia inflata*). Because the effects of lobelia on your body are similar to those of nicotine, lobelia is sometimes recommended as an aid to quitting smoking. Although there have been no reported interactions between lobelia and nicotine, combining the two could increase the risks of nicotine side effects such as dizziness, fatigue, irritability, dry mouth, and headaches. Use lobelia cautiously and only under the supervision of a doctor.
Bear in Mind:	Do not eat or drink anything just before, while, or just after you chew nicotine gum. Caffeine, soft drinks, fruit juice, and wine can block your absorption of nicotine.

Adalat, Procardia

NIFEDIPINE

Type of Drug:	Calcium channel blocker
Description:	Nifedipine, prescribed for high blood pressure and angina, is a calcium channel blocker, a drug that causes blood vessels to relax and widen.
Don't Mix With:	No known herbal interactions.
Bear in Mind:	A substance in grapefruit or grapefruit juice may cause the liver to reduce the rate of elimination of nifedipine. This can increase the amount of the drug in your body to dangerous levels. Avoid grapefruit and grapefruit juice when taking nifedipine.

Furadantin, Macrobid, Macrodantin

NITROFURANTOIN

Type of Drug:	Urinary tract antiinfective
Description:	Nitrofurantoin is prescribed to treat bacterial urinary tract infections, including cystitis. Nitrofurantoin can cause liver damage when taken with oral antidiabetes drugs such as glipizide (see page 83) or glyburide (see page 84). It can also interact adversely with some antibiotics and other drugs. Be certain to tell your doctor about all prescription and nonprescription drugs and dietary supplements you take.
Don't Mix With:	No known herbal interactions.
Bear in Mind:	The magnesium in many nonprescription antacids reduces the amount of nitrofurantoin you absorb. Ask your doctor or pharmacist to recommend a different kind of antacid. Long-term use of nitrofurantoin could block your absorption of folic acid (folate). Consider taking supplements (400 mcg daily) taken at least two hours apart from the drug. Take nitrofurantoin with food to improve absorption and avoid stomach upset.

This drug is sold only in generic form.

NITROGLYCERIN

Type of Drug:	Antianginal drug
Description:	Nitroglycerin is a very powerful drug used to treat angina and chest pain. It is also used to treat heart failure and high blood pressure.
Don't Mix With:	Caffeine-containing herbs. Because caffeine acts as a stimulant and can raise your blood pressure and increase your heart rate, do not use it if taking nitroglycerin. Avoid caffeine-containing herbs, including guaraná (*Paullinia cupana*), kola nut (*Cola spp.*), and maté (*Ilex paraguariensis*). Ephedra (*Ephedra spp.*, also known as ma huang). Taking the stimulant herb ephedra when taking nitroglycerin raises your risk of dangerous high blood pressure and heart arrhythmias. Similarly, avoid the drugs ephedrine and pseudoephedrine, which are found in many nonprescription cold and allergy remedies. Yohimbe (*Pausinystalia yohimbe*). This dangerous herb is sometimes used for erectile dysfunction; one of its side effects is a sharp increase in blood pressure. Never use yohimbe if you are taking nitroglycerin.
Bear in Mind:	Do not combine nitroglycerin and alcohol. Serious and possibly fatal side effects, such as a rapid drop in blood pressure, may occur. The stimulant effect of caffeine may be dangerous when combined with nitroglycerin. If taking this drug, avoid caffeine-containing products and drinks including coffee, tea, cola drinks, many soft drinks, and certain "energy-boosting" products.

Generic only

NITROUS OXIDE

Type of Drug:	Anesthetic gas
Description:	Nitrous oxide, also known as laughing gas, is an anesthetic gas sometimes used during dental work and surgery. When used during dental work, nitrous oxide causes deep relaxation; when used for surgery, it causes deep relaxation or unconsciousness. In general, nitrous oxide is used as a surgical anesthetic only if the patient can't be given other anesthetic drugs. If you take prescription drugs or have a chronic health problem and plan to have nitrous oxide for dental work, discuss it with your doctor and your dentist first.
Don't Mix With:	Sedative herbs. Do not use sedative herbs within 48 hours before or after using nitrous oxide; you may become overly sedated. Avoid sedative herbs such as chamomile (*Matricaria recutita*), catnip (*Nepeta cataria*), kava kava (*Piper methysticum*), passionflower (*Passiflora incarnata*), St. John's wort (*Hypericum perforatum*), valerian (*Valeriana officinalis*), and others, as well as sedative dietary supplements such as 5-HTP, tryptophan, and SAMe.
Do Take With:	Ginger (*Zingiber officinale*). Many patients are nauseous or vomit after awakening from nitrous oxide anesthesia. Ginger capsules can help prevent this effect. Discuss ginger with your dentist or doctor and consider taking supplements (1 gram powdered ginger root in capsules 1 hour before anesthesia).

Axid, Axid-AR

NIZATIDINE

Type of Drug:	H2 blocker antacid
Description:	Nizatidine sharply reduces your production of stomach acid. In prescription form (Axid) it is used to treat ulcers and gastroesophageal reflux disease (GERD). In nonprescription form (Axid-AR) it is used for mild heartburn.
Don't Mix With:	No known herbal interactions.
Do Take With:	Deglycyrrhizinated licorice (DGL, derived from *Glycyrrhiza glabra*). DGL can speed ulcer healing as it stimulates the production of mucus that protects the stomach lining and also has an antiinflammatory effect. Consider taking supplements (250 mg two to three times daily).
Bear in Mind:	Nizatidine and other H2 blockers reduce your absorption of a number of vitamins and minerals including folic acid (folate), vitamin B12 (cobalamin), zinc, and iron. If you use these drugs on a regular basis, consider taking a multivitamin and mineral supplement, along with additional folic acid (400 mcg daily) and vitamin B12 (500 mcg daily). Take these supplements at least two hours apart from nizatidine. Magnesium supplements and calcium-, magnesium-, and magnesium/aluminum-based antacids may block your absorption of nizatidine. Take them at least two hours apart from this drug.

Prilosec

OMEPROZOLE

Type of Drug:	Proton pump inhibitor antacid
Description:	Omeprazole "turns off" your production of stomach acid. It is used to treat ulcers, severe heartburn, and gastroesophageal reflux disease (GERD).
Don't Mix With:	No known herbal interactions.
Do Take With:	Deglycyrrhizinated licorice (DGL, derived from *Glycyrrhiza glabra*). DGL can speed ulcer healing as it stimulates the production of mucus that protects the stomach lining and also has an anti-inflammatory effect. Consider supplements (250 mg two to three times daily).
Bear in Mind:	Omeprazole may block your absorption of certain vitamins and minerals, particularly folic acid (folate), vitamin B12 (cobalamin) and iron. If you use omeprazole or another proton pump inhibitor on a regular basis, take a multivitamin supplement with minerals at least two hours apart from taking the drug, and additional folic acid (400 mcg daily) and vitamin B12 (500 mcg daily).

Alesse, Brevicon, Genora, Loestrin, Necon, Ortho-Novum, others

ORAL CONTRACEPTIVES

Type of Drug:	Contraceptive
Description:	Oral contraceptives are used to prevent pregnancy. They usually contain a mixture of the female hormones estrogen and progesterone (see page 132) in synthetic form; some types contain only progestin (progesterone). A number of prescription drugs can interact adversely with oral contraceptives or make them less effective. Be certain to tell your doctor about all drugs and supplements you take.
Don't Mix With: 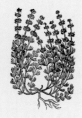	Caffeine-containing herbs. It is possible that consuming large amounts of caffeine may reduce the effectiveness. Discuss your intake of caffeine-containing herbs, such as guaraná (*Paullinia cupana*), kola nut (*Cola spp.*), and maté (*Ilex paraguariensis*), as well as other caffeine-containing, with your medical practitioner. Estrogenic herbs. The herbs black cohosh (*Cimicifuga racemosa*), chaste tree (*Vitex agnus-castus*), dong quai (*Angelica sinensis*), red clover (*Trifolium pratense*), and the supplement soy isoflavones all have estrogenic or estrogen-like effects. Do not use them in combination with oral contraceptives, as contraceptive failure could occur. Other estrogen- and progesterone-modulating herbs. Laboratory studies have shown that the herbs damiana (*Ternera diffusa Willdenow*), hops (*Humulus lupuus*), licorice (*Glycyrrhiza glabra*), oregano (*Origanum vulgare*), thyme (*Thymus spp.*), turmeric (*Curcuma longa*), and vervain (*Verbena spp.*) may modulate estrogen and/or progesterone activity. Discuss the use of these herbs with your doctor before taking an oral contraceptive. St. John's wort (*Hypericum perforatum*). Some women report irregular bleeding when combining this herb with oral contraceptives. Until more is known, don't use it with oral contraceptives, without discussing with your doctor.

Daypro

OXAPROZIN

Type of Drug:	Nonsteroidal antiinflammatory drug (NSAID)
Description:	Oxaprozin is prescribed to treat pain and swelling from arthritis.
Don't Mix With:	Photo-sensitizing herbs. Oxaprozin may make your skin extremely sensitive to sunlight. Because St. John's wort (*Hypericum perforatum*) and dong quai (*Angelica sinensis*) also have this effect when taken for more than a few days, don't combine the drug with these herbs. Avoid direct sun and wear sunscreen. Salicylate-containing herbs. Taking these herbs with oxaprozin could cause severe side effects, including gastrointestinal bleeding. The herbs meadowsweet (*Filipendula ulmaria*), white willow bark (*Salix alba*), and wintergreen (*Gaultheria procumbens*) contain salicylates, a chemical similar to aspirin (another NSAID).
Do Take With:	Deglycyrrhizinated licorice (DGL, derived from *Glycyrrhiza glabra*) stimulates the production of mucus that protects the stomach lining and also has an antiinflammatory effect. It may help prevent the stomach irritation often caused by oxaprozin. Consider taking supplements (400 mg 2 to 4 times daily).
Bear In Mind:	Oxaprozin can raise the amount of potassium in your body. Avoid potassium supplements or salt substitutes while taking this drug. Discuss your intake of valerian (*Valeriana officinalis*), and others, as well as sedative dietary supplements such as 5-HTP, tryptophan, and SAMe, with your doctor. Oxycodone causes drowsiness, impaired judgment, and loss of coordination. Alcohol makes these side effects worse. Don't use alcohol if taking this drug. To prevent constipation, a common side effect of codeine, eat plenty of fresh fruits and vegetables and whole grains and drink plenty of water (at least 64 ounces a day).

Percodan, Percocet, Roxicet, Roxiprin, others

OXYCODONE

Type of Drug:	Narcotic analgesic
Description:	Oxycodone is a narcotic drug made from codeine. In combination with acetaminophen (see page 11) or aspirin (see page 22), oxycodone is prescribed to relieve moderate to severe pain.
Don't Mix With:	Sedative herbs. When combined with oxycodone these herbs may cause excessive drowsiness. Avoid sedative herbs such as chamomile (*Matricaria recutita*), catnip (*Nepeta cataria*), kava kava (*Piper methysticum*), passionflower (*Passiflora incarnata*), St. John's wort (*Hypericum perforatum*), valerian (*Valeriana officinalis*), and others, as well as sedative dietary supplements such as 5-HTP, tryptophan, and SAMe.
Bear in Mind:	Oxycodone causes drowsiness, impaired judgment, and loss of coordination. Alcohol makes these side effects worse. Don't use alcohol if taking this drug. To prevent constipation, a common side effect of codeine, eat plenty of fresh fruits and vegetables and whole grains and drink plenty of water (at least 64 ounces a day).

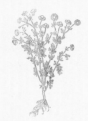

Taxol

PACLITAXEL

Type of Drug:	Anticancer
Description:	Paclitaxel is a chemotherapy drug made from a type of yew tree. It is used to treat ovarian cancer, breast cancer, Kaposi's sarcoma, and a wide range of other cancers. Patients receiving paclitaxel are usually also given other drugs to help relieve or prevent side effects. Be sure to tell your medical practitioner about any prescription or nonprescription drugs and supplements you are taking.
Don't Mix With:	No known herbal interactions.
Bear in Mind:	Although studies are very preliminary, it is possible that the amino acid glutamine could help reduce the side effects of paclitaxel, especially muscle and joint pain. Discuss glutamine with your doctor and consider taking supplements (10 grams three times daily, starting 24 hours after paclitaxel administration and continuing for five to ten days). B vitamins can help prevent or relieve neuropathy (nerve pain and tingling) from paclitaxel. Discuss this with your medical practitioner and consider supplements (B-50 formula once daily). The dietary supplement lipoic acid may also help neuropathy. Discuss this with your doctor and consider supplements (200 mg daily).

Protonix

PANTOPROZOLE

Type of Drug:	Proton pump inhibitor
Description:	Pantoprazole "turns off" your production of stomach acid. It is used to treat ulcers, severe heartburn, and gastroesophageal reflux disease (GERD).
Don't Mix With:	No known herbal interactions.
Do Take With:	Deglycyrrhizinated licorice (DGL, derived from *Glycyrrhiza glabra*). DGL can speed ulcer healing as it stimulates the production of mucus that protects the stomach lining and it also has an anti-inflammatory effect. Consider supplements (250 mg two to three times daily).
Bear in Mind:	Pantoprazole may block your absorption of certain vitamins and minerals, particularly folic acid (folate), vitamin B12 (cobalamin), and iron. If you use pantoprazole or other proton pump inhibitors on a regular basis, take a multivitamin supplement with minerals at least two hours apart from taking the drug, and additional folic acid (400 mcg daily) and vitamin B12 (500 mcg daily).

Paxil

PAROXETINE

Type of Drug:	Selective serotonin reuptake inhibitor (SSRI); antidepressant
Description:	Paroxetine is used to treat depression, obsessive-compulsive disorder, social phobias, panic disorder, and post-traumatic stress syndrome. Like all SSRI drugs, paroxetine affects the way your body uses the neurotransmitter serotonin.
Don't Mix With:	Sedative herbs. When combined with paroxetine these herbs may cause excessive drowsiness. Avoid sedative herbs such as chamomile (*Matricaria recutita*), catnip (*Nepeta cataria*), kava kava (*Piper methysticum*), passionflower (*Passiflora incarnata*), valerian (*Valeriana officinalis*), and others.
	St. John's wort (*Hypericum perforatum*). Although there have been no reports of dangerous interactions, it is possible that combining this herb with paroxetine could raise your serotonin levels too high. If you wish to take St. John's wort instead of paroxetine, discuss it with your doctor.
Do Take With:	Ginkgo (*Ginkgo biloba*). Sexual dysfunction in both men and women is a fairly common side effect of paroxetine. Ginkgo may be helpful for this problem. Consider supplements (60 mg ginkgo extract standardized to 24% ginkgo flavone glycosides three times daily).
Bear in Mind:	Paroxetine can cause drowsiness and dizziness. Alcohol can make these side effects worse. Don't use it when taking this drug. Don't use the dietary supplements 5-HTP, tryptophan, or SAMe if you take paroxetine. They may cause your serotonin level to rise too high.

Cuprimine, Depen

PENICILLAMINE

Type of Drug:	Chelating agent
Description:	Penicillamine is used to treat severe rheumatoid arthritis, Wilson's disease, and cystinuria.
Don't Mix With:	No known herbal interactions.
Bear in Mind:	Penicillamine binds to the minerals copper, iron, magnesium, and zinc in your digestive tract; this prevents you from absorbing both the minerals and the drug. If you are taking penicillamine for rheumatoid arthritis, consider taking a daily multivitamin with m inerals. Take the supplement two hours apart from the drug. If you are taking penicillamine for Wilson's disease, do not take copper supplements in any form. Penicillamine promotes excretion of vitamin B6 (pyridoxine), consider taking supplements (50 mg daily).

Betapen-VK, Pen-Vee K, Pfizerpen, V-Cillin K, Veetids, others

PENICILLIN

Type of Drug:	Antibiotic
Description:	Penicillin is an antibiotic that kills bacteria that cause infections.
Don't Mix With:	No known herbal interactions.
Bear in Mind:	Bromelain, an enzyme found in pineapples, increases your absorption of penicillin. This may be helpful for people with severe infections or infections that don't respond to penicillin. Discuss bromelain supplements with your doctor.
	Penicillin kills not only the harmful bacteria that cause illness but also the good bacteria that are normally found in your intestines; this can cause diarrhea. Consider probiotic supplements (at least 1.5 billion live organisms daily, including a mixture of *Lactobacillus acidophilus, Bifidobacterium bifidum*, and *Saccharomyces boulardii*).
	Drink fruit juices and carbonated beverages at least two hours apart from when you take penicillin. The acid in these drinks decreases activity of the drug before it can get into your bloodstream.

Nardil

PHENELZINE SULFATE

Type of Drug:	Monoamine oxidase (MAO) inhibitor antidepressant
Description:	Phenelzine is an MAO inhibitor prescribed to treat depression, especially depression that doesn't respond to other drugs. Foods that contain a substance called tyramine can cause a dangerous interaction with MAO inhibitors (see *Bear in Mind section*), as can a number of other drugs.
Don't Mix With:	Ephedra (*Ephedra spp.*, also known as ma huang). Taking ephedra with phenelzine raises your risk of serious high blood pressure and heart arrhythmias. Similarly, avoid the drugs ephedrine (see page 71) and pseudoephedrine (see page 136), which are found in many nonprescription cold and allergy remedies. Ginseng (*Panax ginseng*). There have been a few reports of a variety of adverse interactions between ginseng and phenelzine. Until more is known, avoid ginseng. St. John's wort (*Hypericum perforatum*). Research suggests that this herb and phenelzine work in similar ways. To avoid increasing the effect of the drug, don't take St. John's wort. Scotch broom (*Cytisus scoparius*). This herb, sometimes used to treat heart arrhythmias, contains a high amount of tyramine (see below). Don't use it with phenelzine.
Bear in Mind:	Combining phenelzine with tyramine, an amino acid found in many foods, can cause diarrhea, vasodilation (flushing), and dangerous changes in blood pressure, among other symptoms. Foods high in tyramine include alcohol, cheese, fava beans, fermented foods such as sauerkraut and miso soup, bologna, pepperoni, liver, pickled herring, yeast and protein supplements, and caffeine. Discuss food restrictions with your doctor and follow them carefully. Phenelzine may increase the effect of the amino acid tryptophan, sold as 5-HTP. This could cause excessive drowsiness.

Dimetapp, DayQuil Allergy Relief, Tavist-D., Dexatrim, others

PHENYLPROPANOLAMINE

Type of Drug:	Antihistamine
Description:	Phenylpropanolamine is a nonprescription antihistamine (Propagest, Rhindecon, others) used to relieve nasal congestion from colds, sinusitis, and seasonal allergies. In combination with other drugs such as brompheniramine (Dimetapp, DayQuil Allergy Relief, others), chlorpheniramine (Contac 12 Hour, Triaminic, others), and clemastine (Tavist-D), phenylpropanolamine is used to treat cold and allergy symptoms. In combination with drugs such as dextromethorphan (Robitussin CF, others), it is used to relieve coughing. Because appetite loss is a side effect of phenylpropanolamine, it is also used as a nonprescription drug for short-term weight loss (Acutrim, Dexatrim, Unitrol, others).
Don't Mix With:	Ephedra (*Ephedra spp.*, also known as ma huang). The effects and side effects of phenylpropanolamine are similar to those of the stimulant herb ephedra. Combining the two could raise your blood pressure too high and might cause heart arrhythmias. Similarly, avoid the drugs ephedrine (see page 71) and pseudoephedrine (see page 136), which are found in many nonprescription cold and allergy remedies. Caffeine-containing herbs. The stimulant effect of caffeine could interact adversely with phenylpropanolamine. Avoid caffeine-containing herbs, including guaraná (*Paullinia cupana*), kola nut (*Cola spp.*), and maté (*Ilex paraguariensis*).
Bear in Mind:	Caffeine's stimulant effect could cause an adverse reaction if taken with phenylpropanolamine. Coffee, tea, and cola drinks naturally contain caffeine; it is also added to many soft drinks and "energy-boosting" products. Avoid these if taking phenylpropanolamine.

Dilantin

PHENYTOIN

Type of Drug:	Antiepileptic
Description:	Phenytoin is prescribed to treat epilepsy. It is also used to treat some heart rhythm problems.
Don't Mix With:	Caffeine-containing herbs. Phenytoin can cause nervousness, insomnia, confusion, and irritability. To avoid worsening these effects, avoid caffeine-containing herbs, including guaraná (*Paullinia cupana*), kola nut (*Cola spp.*), and maté (*Ilex paraguariensis*), as well as drinks and other products that contain caffeine. Ephedra (*Ephedra spp.*, also known as ma huang). Some side effects of phenytoin, including insomnia and nervousness, may be exacerbated by the stimulant herb ephedra. Do not use it if taking this drug. Similarly, avoid the drugs ephedrine (see page 71) and pseudo-ephedrine (see page 136), which are found in many nonprescription cold and allergy drugs.
Bear in Mind:	B vitamin supplements, especially vitamin B6 (pyridoxine) decrease the effectiveness of phenytoin. Phenytoin, however, also blocks your absorption of B vitamins, especially folic acid (folate), to the point that supplements are usually prescribed to avoid deficiency. Discuss B vitamin supplements with your doctor—you will need to be monitored to make sure you have the correct levels of both the vitamins and phenytoin. Take B vitamin supplements at least two hours apart from this drug. Phenytoin can interfere with your body's absorption of calcium, which may lead to osteoporosis. Discuss calcium and vitamin D (needed for calcium absorption) supplements with your doctor. When using calcium supplements, take them two hours apart from phenytoin; they may slow absorption of the drug. Pregnant women who take phenytoin may need supplements to prevent vitamin K deficiency in their babies. Discuss vitamin K and all other supplements with your doctor.

Kaochlor, K-Dur, Klorvess, K-Lyte/Cl, Slow-K, many others

POTASSIUM CHLORIDE

Type of Drug:	Electrolyte replacement
Description:	Potassium chloride is most commonly prescribed for people who are taking a diuretic, such as furosemide (see page 80), which causes increased excretion of potassium. Note that potassium chloride is also an ingredient in many salt substitutes.
Don't Mix With: 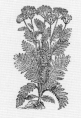	Diuretic herbs. These could cause the elimination of more potassium than you get from supplements and food, especially if you also take a prescription diuretic. Avoid herbal diuretics including bilberry leaf (*Vaccinium myrtillus*), buchu (*Barosma betulina*), burdock (*Arctium lappa*), couch grass (*Agropyron repens*), damiana (*Turnera diffusa*), dandelion (*Taraxacum officinale*), fennel seed (*Foeniculum vulgare*), goldenrod (*Solidago virgaurea*), horsetail (*Equisetum arvense*), kava kava (*Piper methysticum*), kola nut (*Cola spp.*), marshmallow (*Althaea officinalis*), maté (*Ilex paraguariensis*), parsley (*Petroselinum spp.*), sarsaparilla (*Smilax spp.*), saw palmetto (*Serenoa repens*), uva ursi (*Arctostaphylos uva ursi*), vervain (*Verbena spp.*), and yarrow (*Achillea millefolium*), and other herbal and nonprescription diuretics. Licorice (*Glycyrrhiza glabra*). This herb can raise your blood pressure to dangerous levels, especially in combination with potassium supplements. Although deglycyrrhizinated licorice (DGL), a supplement sometimes used to prevent or treat ulcers and stomach irritation, does not contain the ingredient that raises blood pressure, it may still have an effect in combination with potassium supplements and should be avoided.
Bear in Mind:	If your doctor has prescribed a potassium supplement, do not use salt substitutes – you could take in too much potassium. Many fruits and vegetables, and a number of other foods, are high in potassium. Discuss with your doctor.

Pravachol

PRAVASTATIN

Type of Drug:	Statin cholesterol-lowering agent
Description:	Pravastatin is prescribed to lower high cholesterol, slow or prevent hardening of the arteries, and reduce the risk of heart attack and stroke.
Don't Mix With:	No known herbal interactions.
Do Take With:	Milk thistle (*Silybum marianum*). Pravastatin can cause liver damage. Silymarin, the active compound in milk thistle, may prevent or reduce the damage. Consider taking milk thistle supplements (150 mg three to four times daily).
Bear in Mind:	Lovastatin, a drug similar to pravastatin, interacts adversely with grapefruit juice. There are no studies yet of pravastatin and grapefruit juice, but similar problems are possible. Until more is known, do not take pravastatin with grapefruit juice. The dietary supplement red yeast rice, sold as Cholestin, works in a way similar to the statin drugs. Do not use red yeast rice with pravastatin. According to one study, statin drugs can gradually raise your vitamin A level. Until more is known, don't take vitamin A supplements with pravastatin. Several studies show that taking statin drugs can significantly lower your level of coenzyme Q10 (CoQ10 or ubiquinone), a substance needed for energy production in your cells. Consider taking supplements (100 mg daily). Two recent studies suggest that moderate doses of niacin (500 mg twice daily) along with pravastatin lowers cholesterol significantly more than taking the drug alone. Discuss niacin with your doctor before you try it, however, because high doses of niacin interact adversely with some statin drugs.

PREDNISONE

Type of Drug:	Corticosteroid
Description:	Corticosteroids such as prednisone are synthetic hormones used to treat a wide variety of severe disorders, particularly those that involve inflammation, including arthritis, psoriasis, allergies, asthma, and inflammatory bowel disease. Corticosteroids are also used to treat autoimmune diseases such as lupus erythematosus and transplant rejection.
Don't Mix With:	Digitalis (*Digitalis spp.*, also known as foxglove). This dangerous herb is very similar to the heart drug digoxin (see page 61), which may worsen side effects of prednisone. Digitalis may cause the same problem. Ephedra (*Ephedra spp.*, also known as ma huang). The herb ephedra naturally contains ephedrine, which can reduce the effectiveness of corticosteroids. Do not use it when taking prednisone. Similarly, avoid the drugs ephedrine (see page 71) and pseudoephedrine (see page 136), which are found in many nonprescription cold and allergy remedies.
Bear in Mind:	Long-term use of corticosteroids may cause osteoporosis, probably because the drug interferes with your use of calcium and vitamin D. Studies have shown that taking supplements helps prevent corticosteroid-induced osteoporosis. Consider taking supplements (1,000 mg calcium daily, 400 IU vitamin D daily). Corticosteroids may also reduce your level of vitamin B6 (pyridoxine) and magnesium. Consider supplements (50 mg pyroxidine and 300–400 mg magnesium daily). Long term use of corticosteroids reduces your level of chromium, which may contribute to the development of diabetes. Consider taking supplements (200 mcg chromium picolinate daily).

Amen, Crinone, Cycrin, Curretab, Depo-Provera, Prometrium, Provera

PROGESTERONE

Type of Drug:	Progestin
Description:	Progesterone (often in the semisynthetic form medoxyprogesterone) is prescribed to treat irregular menstrual bleeding, endometriosis, premenstrual syndrome (PMS), and some other problems. Combined with estrogen or in conjugated estrogens (see page 52), it is used to treat menopause symptoms such as hot flashes. It is also used to treat sleep apnea and in formulations that prevent pregnancy.
Don't Mix With:	Progesterone-modulating herbs. Laboratory studies have shown that the herbs damiana (*Turnera diffusa*), oregano (*Origanum vulgare*), red clover (*Trifolium pratense*), thyme (*Thyme spp.*), turmeric (*Curcuma longa*), and vervain (*Verbena spp.*) may modulate progesterone activity. Discuss the use of these herbs with your medical practitioner before using them if you take progesterone.

Phenergan, others

PROMETHAZINE

Type of Drug:	Antihistamine
Description:	Promethazine is an antihistamine used to treat seasonal allergies, motion sickness, and nausea and vomiting. In combination with codeine (see page 50) or dextromethorphan (see page 57), promethazine is used in prescription and nonprescription syrup cough remedies.
Don't Mix With:	Henbane (*Hyoscyamus niger*). This herb is toxic and should be used only when prescribed and closely monitored by a qualified practitioner. Because it has side effects similar to those of promethazine, such as heart palpitations, do not use it.
	Sedative herbs. Promethazine has a tranquilizing effect that can be heightened when taken in combination with sedative herbs such as such as German chamomile (*Matricaria recutita*), catnip (*Nepeta cataria*), kava kava (*Piper methysticum*), passionflower (*Passiflora incarnata*), St. John's wort (*Hypericum perforatum*), valerian (*Valeriana officinalis*), and others, as well as sedative dietary supplements such as 5-HTP, tryptophan, and SAMe.
Bear in Mind:	Promethazine often causes drowsiness and dizziness. Alcohol can make these side effects worse. Don't use it if taking this drug. Long-term use of promethazine may increase your need for riboflavin (vitamin B2). Consider taking supplements (a B-50 formula daily).

Darvon, Darvocet

PROPOXYPHENE

Type of Drug:	Narcotic analgesic
Description:	Propoxyphene is a prescription drug used to relieve mild to moderate pain. It is used by itself or combined with a nonsteroidal anti-inflammatory drug such as aspirin (see page 22) or acetaminophen (see page 11); caffeine is also found in some formulas. Propoxyphene is potentially addictive and must be used with caution.
	The antacid cimetidine (see page 41) may cause serious side effects when taken with propoxyphene. Discuss alternative antacids with your medical practitioner or pharmacist.
Don't Mix With:	Sedative herbs. When combined with propoxyphene, these herbs may cause excessive drowsiness. Avoid sedative herbs such as chamomile (*Matricaria recutita*), catnip (*Nepeta cataria*), kava kava (*Piper methysticum*), passionflower (*Passiflora incarnata*), St. John's wort (*Hypericum perforatum*), valerian (*Valeriana officinalis*), and others, as well as sedative dietary supplements such as 5-HTP, tryptophan, and SAMe.
Bear in Mind:	Propoxyphene causes drowsiness. Alcohol makes this side effect worse. Don't use alcohol if taking this drug.
	To avoid constipation, a common side effect of propoxyphene, eat plenty of high-fiber foods, such as fresh fruits and vegetables and whole grains, and drink 64 ounces of water daily.

Inderal

PROPRANOLOL HYDROCHLORIDE

Type of Drug:	Beta blocker

Description: Propranolol is used to treat high blood pressure, angina, and abnormal heart rhythms, and to help prevent a second heart attack. It is also sometimes used to treat bleeding from the stomach or esophagus, migraines, and the symptoms of hyperthyroidism (overactive thyroid gland). In some cases propranolol is used to treat anxiety disorders, schizophrenia, and the side effects of antipsychotic drugs. Propranolol is a powerful drug that can interact adversely with a number of prescription drugs, so use it with caution. Be certain to tell your doctor about any other prescription and nonprescription drugs and dietary supplements you take.

Don't Mix With: 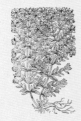 Black pepper (*Piper nigrum*). One study in 1991 suggests that piperine, a chemical found in black pepper, could raise the level of propranolol. Until more is known, avoid eating large amounts of black pepper.

St. John's wort (*Hypericum perforatum*). Monoamine oxidase inhibitors (MAOI drugs) interact adversely with propranolol. Because St. John's wort works in a way similar to these drugs, don't use it if taking propranolol.

Bear in Mind: Beta blockers block your use of coenzyme Q10 (CoQ10 or ubiquinone), which is needed for energy production within your cells. Consider taking supplements (100 mg daily).

The antacid cimetidine (see page 41) increases the amount of propranolol in your bloodstream. Choose a different type of antacid.

Actifed, Afrin, Benadryl, Contac, Sinarest, Sudafed, others

PSEUDOEPHEDRINE

Type of Drug:	Decongestant
Description:	Pseudoephedrine is a nonprescription decongestant that is sold by itself (Afrin, Sudafed, others) or in combination with antihistamines and other medications (Benadryl, Contac, others) to treat seasonal allergies and symptoms of colds and flu.
Don't Mix With:	Caffeine-containing herbs. The stimulant effect of caffeine can make the side effects of pseudoephedrine, such as nervousness, restlessness, insomnia, and dizziness, worse. Avoid caffeine-containing herbs, including guaraná (*Paullinia cupana*), kola nut (*Cola spp.*), and maté (*Ilex paraguariensis*). Ephedra (*Ephedra spp.*, also known as ma huang). Ephedrine, a drug closely related to pseudoephedrine, was originally isolated from ephedra. Taking ephedra with any product containing pseudoephedrine could increase the side effects of the drug, including nervousness, insomnia, dizziness, high blood pressure, and heart arrhythmias. Tannin-containing herbs. Herbs that are high in tannin, including black walnut (*Juglans nigra*), red raspberry (*Rubus idaeus*), oak (*Quercus spp.*), uva ursi (*Arctostaphylos uva ursi*), and witch hazel (*Hamamelis virginiana*), can interfere with your absorption of pseudoephedrine, as can the tannins in tea. Don't consume these substances within two hours of taking this drug.
Bear in Mind:	The side effects of pseudoephedrine, such as nervousness, restlessness, insomnia, and dizziness, may be worsened by caffeine's stimulant effect. Coffee, tea, and cola drinks naturally contain caffeine; it is also added to many soft drinks and "energy-boosting" products. Avoid these when taking ephedrine.

Fiberall, Konsyl, Metamucil, others

PSYLLIUM

Type of Drug:	Bulk laxative
Description:	Psyllium (*Plantago spp.*) is a plant-based form of soluble fiber used to treat occasional constipation by increasing the bulk and softness of the stool. People with asthma have occasionally had asthma attacks from inhaling psyllium dust or using psyllium products. If you have asthma, discuss psyllium with your doctor.
Don't Mix With:	Herbal laxatives. Aloe (*Aloe spp.*), buckthorn (*Rhamnus catharticus*), cascara sagrada (*Rhamnus purshianus*), frangula (*Rhamnus frangula*), also known as buckthorn bark, rhubarb (*Rheum spp.*), and senna (*Cassia spp.*) are powerful laxatives that should be used only when psyllium hasn't helped. When combined with psyllium they can cause diarrhea and cramping.
Bear in Mind:	Frequent use of psyllium can reduce your absorption of many drugs, herbs, and dietary supplements by moving them through your digestive system too quickly. If you must take psyllium on a regular basis, separate it from your other medications and supplements by at least three hours.

Zantac, Zantac 75

RANITIDINE

Type of Drug:	H2 blocker antacid
Description:	Ranitidine sharply reduces your production of stomach acid. In prescription form (Zantac) it is used to treat ulcers and gastroesophageal reflux disease (GERD) and to help prevent internal bleeding from large doses of nonsteroidal anti-inflammatory drugs such as aspirin (see page 22). In nonprescription form (Zantac 75) it is used for mild heartburn.
Don't Mix With:	No known herbal interactions.
Do Take With:	Deglycyrrhizinated licorice (DGL, derived from *Glycyrrhiza glabra*). DGL can speed ulcer healing as it stimulates the production of mucus that protects the stomach lining and also has an antiinflammatory effect. Consider taking supplements (250 mg two to three times daily).
Bear in Mind:	Ranitidine and other H2 blockers reduce your absorption of a number of vitamins and minerals including folic acid (folate), vitamin B12 (cobalamin), zinc, and iron. If you use these drugs on a regular basis, consider taking a multivitamin and mineral supplement, along with additional folic acid (400 mcg daily) and vitamin B12 (500 mcg daily). Take these supplements at least two hours apart from ranitidine. Magnesium supplements and calcium-, magnesium-, and magnesium/aluminum-based antacids may block your absorption of ranitidine. Take them at least two hours apart from ranitidine.

Vioxx

ROFECOXIB

Type of Drug:	Cyclooxygenase-2 (COX-2) inhibitor nonsteroidal antiinflammatory drug (NSAID)
Description:	COX-2 inhibitors are used to treat arthritis. They work by blocking your production of an enzyme that regulates pain and inflammation. COX-2 inhibitors are slightly less likely than are other NSAIDs to cause stomach irritation; they also don't thin your blood like other NSAIDS do. Rofecoxib is also used to treat painful menstruation and acute pain.
Don't Mix With:	Salicylate-containing herbs. In combination with rofecoxib, these herbs could cause severe stomach irritation. They include meadowsweet (*Filipendula ulmaria*), white willow bark (*Salix alba*), and wintergreen (*Gaultheria procumbens*).
Do Take With:	Milk thistle (*Silybum marianum*). Silymarin, the active compound in the herb milk thistle, may help protect your liver against irritation caused by rofecoxib. Consider taking supplements (150 mg three to four times daily).
Bear in Mind:	Many NSAIDs reduce your absorption of folic acid (folate). Although there is no evidence that rofecoxib does this, consider taking supplements (400 mcg daily).

Zoloft

SERTRALINE

Type of Drug:	Selective serotonin reuptake inhibitor (SSRI) antidepressant
Description:	Sertraline is used to treat depression and obsessive-compulsive disorder. Like all SSRI drugs, sertraline affects the way your body uses the neurotransmitter serotonin.
Don't Mix With:	Sedative herbs. When combined with sertraline these herbs may cause excessive drowsiness. Avoid sedative herbs such as chamomile (*Matricaria recutita*), catnip (*Nepeta cataria*), kava kava (*Piper methysticum*), passionflower (*Passiflora incarnata*), valerian (*Valeriana officinalis*), and others.
	St. John's wort (*Hypericum perforatum*). Although there have been no reports of dangerous interactions, it is possible that combining this herb with sertraline could raise your serotonin levels too high. If you wish to take St. John's wort instead of sertraline, discuss it with your doctor.
Do Take With:	Ginkgo (*Ginkgo biloba*). Sexual dysfunction in both men and women is a fairly common side effect of sertraline. Gingko may be helpful for reducing this problem. Consider supplements (60 mg gingko extract standardized to 24% ginkgo flavone glycosides three times daily).
Bear in Mind:	Sertraline can cause drowsiness and dizziness. Alcohol can make these side effects worse. Don't use it if taking this drug.
	Don't use the dietary supplements 5-HTP, tryptophan, or SAMe if you take sertraline. They may cause your serotonin level to rise too high.

Zocor

SIMVASTATIN

Type of Drug:	Statin cholesterol-lowering agent
Description:	Simvastatin is prescribed to lower high cholesterol, slow or prevent hardening of the arteries, and reduce the risk of heart attack and stroke.
Don't Mix With:	No known herbal interactions.
Do Take With:	Milk thistle (*Silybum marianum*). Although there are no studies to date, silymarin, the active compound in the herb milk thistle may protect against the liver damage that can occur as a side effect of this type of drug. Consider taking supplements (150 mg three to four times daily).
Bear in Mind:	Lovastatin, a drug similar to simvastatin, interacts adversely with grapefruit juice. There are no studies yet of simvastatin and grapefruit juice, but similar problems are possible. Until more is known, do not take simvastatin with grapefruit juice. The dietary supplement, red yeast rice, sold as Cholestin, works in a way similar to the statin drugs. Do not use red yeast rice with simvastatin. According to one study, statin drugs can gradually raise vitamin A levels. Until more is known, don't take vitamin A supplements. Several studies show that taking statin drugs can significantly lower your level of coenzyme Q10 (CoQ10 or ubiquinone), a substance needed for energy production in your cells. Consider taking supplements (100 mg daily). Some research suggests that moderate doses of niacin (500 mg twice daily) along with simvastatin could lower cholesterol significantly more than taking the drug alone. Discuss niacin with your doctor before you try it, however, because high doses of niacin interact adversely with some statin drugs.

Bactrim, Gantanol, Septra, others

SULFAMETHOXAZOLE

Type of Drug:	Sulfonamide antibiotic
Description:	Sulfamethoxazole is prescribed by itself (Gantanol) or in combination with another antibiotic drug called trimethoprim (Bactrim, Cotrim, Septra, others). The combination is also known as TMP/SMZ. Both drugs are used to treat infections caused by bacteria or protozoa, especially urinary tract infections.
Don't Mix With:	Salicylate-containing herbs. The herbs meadowsweet (*Filipendula ulmaria*), white willow bark (*Salix alba*), and wintergreen (*Gaultheria procumbens*) contain salicylates, compounds similar to aspirin (see page 22). Do not take them in conjunction with sulfamethoxazole or TMP/SMZ; it could make your salicylate level rise too high. Photo-sensitizing herbs. Sulfamethoxazole can make your skin very sensitive to sun. Because St. John's wort (*Hypericum perforatum*) and dong quai (*Angelica sinensis*) also have this effect when taken for more than a few days, don't combine the drug with these herbs. Avoid direct sun and wear sunscreen.
Bear in Mind:	Both sulfamethoxazole and TMP/SMZ block the body's ability to use or absorb folic acid (folate), vitamin B6 (pyridoxine), and vitamin B12 (cobalamin). If you take these drugs on a long-term basis, consider taking supplements (B-50 formula daily). These drugs also decrease the absorption of calcium and magnesium and may affect the level of vitamin K. Consider taking a daily multivitamin with minerals. Take all vitamin and mineral supplements at least two hours apart from sulfamethoxazole. The dietary supplement PABA may block the action of sulfamethoxazole. Until more is known, do not take PABA supplements when taking this drug. The PABA in sunscreens is unlikely to have any effect on sulfamethoxazole and is safe to use.

Azulfidine

SULFASALAZINE

Type of Drug:	Sulfonamide antibiotic
Description:	Sulfasalazine is prescribed to treat rheumatoid arthritis, ulcerative colitis, and Crohn's disease. Although this drug is a type of antibiotic, it is used because it is also reduces inflammation.

Don't Mix With:

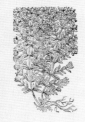

Salicylate-containing herbs. The herbs meadowsweet (*Filipendula ulmaria*), white willow bark (*Salix alba*), and wintergreen (*Gaultheria procumbens*) contain salicylates, compounds similar to aspirin (see page 22). Do not take them in conjunction with sulfasalazine; it could raise salicylate levels too high.

Photo-sensitizing herbs. Sulfasalazine can make your skin very sensitive to sun. Because St. John's wort (*Hypericum perforatum*) and dong quai (*Angelica sinensis*) also have this effect when taken for more than a few days, don't combine the drug with these herbs. Avoid direct sun and wear sunscreen.

Bear in Mind:

The dietary supplement PABA may block the action of sulfasalazine. Until more is known, do not take PABA supplements when taking this drug. The PABA in sunscreens is unlikely to have any effect on sulfasalazine and is safe to use.

Sulfasalazine blocks your absorption of folic acid (folate). Discuss this problem with your doctor and consider taking supplements (800 mcg daily). Take them at least two hours apart from the drug. Iron can bind with sulfasalazine and keep the drug from being absorbed. Take iron supplements two hours apart from sulfasalazine.

Imitrex

SUMATRIPTAN

Type of Drug:	Triptan–type antimigraine
Description:	Sumatriptan is prescribed to help prevent and relieve migraines. It works by affecting serotonin receptors in your brain. Sumatriptan and other triptan drugs should not be used if you have or are at risk for heart disease – heart problems have developed in people using this drug. Triptan drugs can interact adversely with MAO inhibitors such as phenelzine (see page 126) and with other drugs, including birth control pills (see page 118). Be certain to tell your doctor about all prescription and nonprescription drugs and dietary supplements you take.
Don't Mix With:	Feverfew (*Tanacetum parthenium*). Recent studies have shown that the herb feverfew can help prevent migraines. There are no studies showing possible interactions between feverfew and sumatriptan, but you should discuss feverfew with your doctor before you take it with sumatriptan. St. John's wort (*Hypericum perforatum*). St. John's wort and sumatriptan may work in similar ways. Combining them could cause your serotonin levels to become too high. Until more is known, don't take St. John's wort when taking sumatriptan.
Bear in Mind:	The natural sedatives 5-HTP, L-tryptophan, and SAMe all affect your serotonin levels, as does sumatriptan. Don't combine them with this drug.

Nolvadex
TAMOXIFEN

Type of Drug:	Antiestrogen
Description:	Tamoxifen blocks the use of the hormone estrogen. It is used to treat breast cancers that grow more quickly in the presence of estrogen, and to help prevent recurrences. Tamoxifen is also used for some other types of cancer such as pancreatic cancer and endometrial cancer.
Don't Mix With:	Estrogenic herbs. The herbs black cohosh (*Cimicifuga racemosa*), dong quai (*Angelica sinensis*), chaste tree (*Vitex agnus-castus*), and red clover (*Trifolium pratense*) all have estrogen-like effects. Do not use them in combination with tamoxifen.
Do Take With:	Milk thistle (*Silybum marianum*). Silymarin, the active compound in the herb milk thistle, may help protect your liver against irritation caused by tamoxifen. Consider taking supplements (200 mg daily).
Bear in Mind:	Studies in laboratory animals suggest that soy isoflavones (estrogen-like substances) may help tamoxifen work better. The research is controversial, however, and the long-term value of taking soy isoflavones is unknown.
	High doses of melatonin, a natural hormone, may also help tamoxifen work better, especially in patients who are not helped by tamoxifen alone. Discuss both of these supplements with your doctor before trying them.

Ala-Tet, Panmycin, Sumycin, Tetracap, Tetracyn, others

TETRACYCLINE

Type of Drug:	Tetracycline antibiotic
Description:	Tetracycline is prescribed for bacterial infections, including tick-borne infections, acne, and as an alternative antibiotic for people allergic to penicillin.
Don't Mix With:	Berberine-containing herbs. Goldenseal (*Hydrastis canadensis*), barberry (*Berberis vulgaris*), and Oregon grape (*Mahonia spp.*) contain berberine, an antibacterial chemical that may interfere with your absorption of tetracycline. Don't use these herbs when taking tetracycline.
Bear in Mind:	The aluminum, calcium, and magnesium in antacids can interfere with your absorption of tetracycline, as can the calcium, iron, magnesium, zinc, and other minerals in supplements and multivitamins with minerals, and the calcium in milk and other dairy products. Take these antacids and supplements at least two hours apart from tetracycline, and discuss your intake of calcium-rich foods with your medical practitioner. Tetracycline can block your absorption or use of many B vitamins. Consider supplements (B-50 formula once daily). Tetracycline kills not only the harmful bacteria that cause illness but also the good bacteria that are normally found in your intestines; this can cause diarrhea. Consider taking probiotic supplements (at least 1.5 billion live organisms daily, including a mixture of *Lactobacillus acidophilus, Bifidobacterium bifidum*, and *Saccharomyces boulardii*).

Bronkodyl, Slo-bid, Theolair, Theo-Dur, Uniphyl, others

THEOPHYLLINE

Type of Drug:	Bronchodilator
Description:	Theophylline is prescribed to treat asthma and also emphysema, bronchitis, chronic obstructive pulmonary disease (COPD), and some other conditions.
Don't Mix With:	Caffeine-containing herbs. Caffeine can increase the action and side effects of theophylline. Avoid caffeine-containing herbs, including guaraná (*Paullinia cupana*), kola nut (*Cola spp.*), and maté (*Ilex paraguariensis*), and other products that contain caffeine.
	Cayenne (*Capsicum frutescens*). Eating large amounts of cayenne pepper could increase your absorption of theophylline and raise your blood level of this drug too high. Amounts consumed as part of a normal diet are unlikely to cause problems.
	Ephedra (*Ephedra spp.*, also known as ma huang). Taking ephedra with theophylline raises blood pressure and can cause heart arrhythmias and other serious side effects. Similarly, avoid the drugs ephedrine (see page 71) and pseudoephedrine (see page 136), which are found in many nonprescription cold and allergy remedies.
	St. John's wort (*Hypericum perforatum*). This may lower blood levels of theophylline. Until more is known, don't combine these.
	Tannin-containing herbs. Herbs that are high in tannin include black walnut (*Juglans nigra*), red raspberry (*Rubus idaeus*), oak (*Quercus spp.*), uva ursi (*Arctostaphylos uva-ursi*), and witch hazel (*Hamamelis virginiana*). Also tea can interfere with the absorption of theophylline. Do not use these herbs when taking theophylline.
Bear in Mind:	Studies have shown that theophylline depletes vitamin B6 (pyridoxine) levels. Discuss vitamin B6 with your doctor and consider taking supplements (50 mg daily).
	Theophylline may also deplete levels of potassium and magnesium. Discuss supplements with your doctor.

Aquatensen, Diuril, Diurese, Exna, Metahydrin, others

THIAZIDE

Type of Drug:	Potassium-wasting diuretic
Description:	Thiazide diuretics are used most often to treat high blood pressure. These drugs are often called "potassium-wasting" diuretics because they increase elimination of potassium – and also magnesium, sodium, and zinc – from your body.

Don't Mix With:

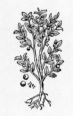

Digitalis (*Digitalis purpurea*, also known as foxglove). This dangerous herb is very similar to the heart drug digoxin, which is derived from digitalis and can lower your potassium level. In combination with a thiazide diuretic, digitalis could make your potassium level dangerously low.

Herbal diuretics. In combination with a thiazide diuretic, herbal diuretics could make your potassium level drop too low. Avoid herbal diuretics, including bilberry leaf (*Vaccinium myrtillus*), buchu (*Barosma betulina*), burdock (*Arctium lappa*), couch grass (*Agropyron repens*), damiana (*Turnera diffusa*), dandelion (*Taraxacum officinale*), fennel seed (*Foeniculum vulgare*), goldenrod (*Solidago virgaurea*), horsetail (*Equisetum arvense*), kava kava (*Piper methysticum*), kola nut (*Cola spp.*), marshmallow (*Althaea officinalis*), maté (*Ilex paraguariensis*), parsley (*Petroselinum spp.*), sarsaparilla (*Smilax spp.*), saw palmetto (*Serenoa repens*), uva ursi (*Arctostaphylos uva ursi*), vervain (*Verbena spp.*), and yarrow (*Achillea millefolium*).

Licorice (*Glycyrrhiza glabra*). Large amounts of licorice can reduce your potassium level. In combination with a thiazide diuretic, this could make your potassium level dangerously low. This effect does not occur with deglycyrrhizinated licorice (DGL) or with artificial licorice flavoring.

Ticlid
TICLOPIDINE

Type of Drug:	Anticoagulant
Description:	Ticlopidine is an anticoagulant ("blood-thinning") drug used to prevent blood clots and reduce the risk of strokes. It is also used to treat intermittent claudication (poor circulation in the legs) and some other conditions, such as sickle cell anemia.

Description:

Ticlopidine is an anticoagulant ("blood-thinning") drug used to prevent blood clots and reduce the risk of strokes. It is also used to treat intermittent claudication (poor circulation in the legs) and some other conditions, such as sickle cell anemia.

H2 antagonist antacids, such as cimetidine (see page 41), slow your elimination of ticlopidine, which raises the amount in your bloodstream and increases the risk of side effects. Ask your doctor or pharmacist to help you choose a different type of antacid.

Don't Mix With:

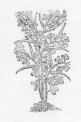

Blood-thinning herbs. A number of herbs have known or possible anticoagulant action and could increase the effect of ticlopidine. Avoid dan shen (*Salvia miltiorrhiza*), devil's claw (*Harpagophytum procumbens*), dong quai (*Angelica sinensis*), fenugreek (*Trigonella foenum-graecum*), garlic (*Allium sativum*), ginger (*Zingiber officinale*), ginkgo (*Ginkgo biloba*), ginseng (*Panax ginseng*), horse chestnut (*Aesculus hippocastanum*), red clover (*Trifolium pratense*), and sweet woodruff (*Galium odoratum*). Foods containing garlic and ginger in moderate amounts are unlikely to cause any problems.

Salicylate-containing herbs. The herbs meadowsweet (*Filipendula ulmaria*), white willow bark (*Salix alba*), and wintergreen (*Gaultheria procumbens*) contain salicylates, compounds similar to aspirin, which can thin the blood. There is a slight chance that taking these herbs with ticlopidine could thin your blood too much.

Bear in Mind:

Magnesium and calcium reduce your absorption of ticlopidine. Take antacids or supplements containing these minerals two hours apart from the drug.

Betimol, Blocadren, Timoptic

TIMOLOL

Type of Drug:	Beta blocker
Description:	Timolol is used to treat high blood pressure and abnormal heart rhythms; it is also used to treat glaucoma. Timolol is a powerful drug that can interact adversely with a number of prescription drugs, so use it with caution. Be certain to tell your doctor about any other prescription and nonprescription drugs and dietary supplements you take.
Don't Mix With:	St. John's wort (*Hypericum perforatum*). Monoamine oxidase inhibitors (MAOI drugs) interact adversely with timolol. Because St. John's wort works in a way that is similar to these drugs, don't use it if taking timolol.
Bear in Mind:	Beta blockers block your use of coenzyme Q10 (CoQ10 or ubiquinone), which is needed for energy production within your cells. Consider taking supplements (20-50 mg daily). The antacid cimetidine (see page 41) and related H2-antagonist antacids such as famotidine (see page 76), and ranitidine (see page 138) may increase the amount of timolol in your bloodstream. Ask your doctor or pharmacist to help you choose a different type of antacid. A small amount of the timolol in eyedrops (Timoptic) enters your bloodstream, but is not enough to cause any of the problems associated with beta blockers.

Ultram
TRAMADOL

Type of Drug:	Nonnarcotic pain reliever
Description:	Tramadol is prescribed to relieve moderate to severe pain.
Don't Mix With:	St. John's wort (*Hypericum perforatum*). Both St. John's wort and tramadol reduce the uptake of serotonin, a neurotransmitter, into your nerves. Combining the two may cause your serotonin level to become too high, which could lead to a serious condition known as serotonin syndrome.
Bear in Mind:	The supplements 5-HTP, L-tryptophan, and SAMe all effect your uptake of serotonin. Don't combine them with tramadol, as your serotonin level may rise too high. Tramadol can cause drowsiness and impair mental ability and coordination. Alcohol can make these side effects worse. Don't use alcohol if taking this drug.

Desyrel

TRAZODONE

Type of Drug:	Antidepressant
Description:	Trazodone is prescribed for depression, panic disorder, agoraphobia (fear of open spaces), and some other disorders. It is also used to treat cocaine addiction.
Don't Mix With:	Digitalis (*Digitalis purpurea*, also known as foxglove). This dangerous herb is very similar to the heart drug digoxin, which, when taken with trazodone, could raise the digoxin in your blood to a dangerous level. Until more is known, don't mix digitalis with trazodone. St. John's wort (*Hypericum perforatum*). Although there have been no reports of interactions, doctors recommend against combining the antidepressant herb St. John's wort with antidepressant drugs such as trazodone.
Bear in Mind:	Trazodone can cause drowsiness and dizziness. Alcohol can make these side effects worse. Don't use alcohol when taking this drug.

Dyazide, Dyrenium, Maxzide

TRIAMTERENE

Type of Drug:	Potassium-sparing diuretic
Description:	Triamterene is a diuretic prescribed alone (Dyrenium) or in combination with hydrochlorothiazide (Dyazide, Maxzide) to treat high blood pressure, heart failure, and some other conditions. Triamterene is a "potassium-sparing" diuretic because it does not cause your body to eliminate excess potassium, in contrast with some other classes of diuretics that are known as "potassium-wasting."
Don't Mix With: 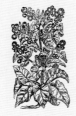	Herbal diuretics. Combining triamterene and diuretic herbs increases the risk of side effects such as electrolyte disturbances and dehydration. Avoid herbal diuretics including bilberry leaf (*Vaccinium myrtillus*), buchu (*Barosma betulina*), burdock (*Arctium lappa*), couch grass (*Agropyron repens*), damiana (*Turnera diffusa*), dandelion (*Taraxacum officinale*), fennel seed (*Foeniculum vulgare*), goldenrod (*Solidago virgaurea*), horsetail (*Equisetum arvense*), kava kava (*Piper methysticum*), kola nut (*Cola nitida*), marshmallow (*Althaea officinalis*), maté (*Ilex paraguariensis*), parsley (*Petroselinum spp.*), sarsaparilla (*Smilax spp.*), saw palmetto (*Serenoa repens*), uva ursi (*Arctostaphylos uva ursi*), vervain (*Verbena spp.*), and yarrow (*Achillea millefolium*), as well as any other prescription or nonprescription diuretics.
Bear in Mind:	Triamterene can increase the amount of potassium in your body. Don't take potassium supplements or use salt substitutes (which are generally high in potassium) with this drug. Discuss your consumption of potassium-rich foods, such as bananas and orange juice, with your doctor. Triamterene might increase your magnesium level. Avoid magnesium supplements and magnesium-containing antacids.

Effexor, Effexor XR

VENLAFAXINE

Type of Drug:	Antidepressant
Description:	Venlafaxine is prescribed to treat depression. Although this drug probably works by reducing the uptake of serotonin, a neurotransmitter, into your nerves, it is not related to selective serotonin reuptake inhibitor (SSRI) drugs such as fluoxetine (see page 77).
Don't Mix With:	St. John's wort (*Hypericum perforatum*). Because St. John's wort is also thought to work by affecting your serotonin levels, don't combine it with venlafaxine. This may cause the level of serotonin in your blood to rise too high, which can result in a serious condition known as serotonin syndrome.
Bear in Mind:	The supplements 5-HTP, L-tryptophan, and SAMe all affect serotonin levels. Don't combine them with venlafaxine as this may cause your serotonin levels to rise too high. Venlafaxine can cause drowsiness and impair mental ability and coordination. Alcohol can make these side effects worse. Don't use alcohol if taking this drug.

Calan, Covera HS, Isoptin, Verelan

VERAPAMIL

Type of Drug:	Calcium channel blocker
Description:	Verapamil is prescribed for high blood pressure, angina, abnormal heart rhythms, and cardiomyopathy. It is also sometimes prescribed to treat nighttime leg cramps, asthma, migraines, and bipolar disorder. Verapamil is a calcium channel blocker, a drug that blocks the movement of calcium into muscles, which allows them to relax, and widens blood vessels.
Don't Mix With:	No known herbal interactions.
Do Take With:	Milk thistle (*Silybum marianum*). Silymarin, the active compound in the herb milk thistle, may help protect against liver damage from verapamil. Consider taking supplements (200 mg daily).
Bear in Mind:	A substance in grapefruit or grapefruit juice may cause the liver to reduce the rate of elimination of other calcium channel blocker drugs such as felodipine (Plendil) and nifedipine (see page 112). This can increase the amount of these drugs in your body to dangerous levels. Although there have been no reports of a similar effect with verapamil, until more is known, don't eat grapefruit or drink grapefruit juice when taking this drug.
	Calcium from supplements or antacids may block the effects of verapamil, and vitamin D may reduce the drug's effectiveness. Discuss any supplements or drugs containing calcium or vitamin D with your medical practitioner.
	To avoid constipation from verapamil, eat plenty of fresh fruits and vegetables and whole grains and drink plenty of water (at least 64 ounces a day).

Coumadin

WARFARIN

Type of Drug:	Anticoagulant
Description:	Warfarin is an anticoagulant ("blood-thinning") drug used primarily to prevent and treat blood clots and to reduce the risk of strokes. Warfarin is a dangerous drug that can interact adversely with a very wide range of other drugs, herbs, vitamins, and other dietary supplements. If at all possible, don't use any herbs, dietary supplements, or nonprescription drugs if taking warfarin. However, if you are taking any herbs, supplements or nonprescription drugs, do not discontinue them until you have discussed it with your doctor.
Don't Mix With:	Blood-thinning herbs. A number of herbs may have anticoagulant action and could increase the effect of warfarin. Avoid dan shen (*Salvia miltiorrhiza*), devil's claw (*Harpagophytum procumbens*), dong quai (*Angelica sinensis*), fenugreek (*Trigonella foenum-graecum*), garlic (*Allium sativum*), ginger (*Zingiber officinale*), ginkgo (*Ginkgo biloba*), ginseng (*Panax ginseng*), horse chestnut (*Aesculus hippocastanum*), red clover (*Trifolium pratense*), and sweet woodruff (*Galium odoratum*). Foods containing garlic and ginger in moderate amounts are unlikely to cause any problems. Salicylate-containing herbs. The herbs meadowsweet (*Filipendula ulmaria*), willow bark (*Salix alba*), and wintergreen (*Gaultheria procumbens*) contain salicylates, compounds similar to aspirin that may also have a blood-thinning effect. Taking these herbs with warfarin could thin your blood too much. St. John's wort (*Hypericum perforatum*). This herb may reduce your absorption of warfarin. Until more is known, don't combine St. John's wort with warfarin.
Bear in Mind:	Warfarin works by blocking your use of vitamin K, which is needed to make your blood clot. Do not take vitamin K supplements with warfarin. Discuss your intake of foods rich in vitamin K with your doctor.

Ambien

ZOLPIDEM

Type of Drug:	Sedative/hypnotic (nonbarbiturate)
Description:	Zolpidem is a sleeping pill prescribed for the short-term treatment of insomnia. Although zolpidem works in ways very similar to benzodiazepine drugs such as diazepam (see page 58), it is not related to these drugs and does not relax muscles.
Don't Mix With: 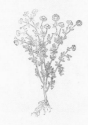	Sedative herbs. When combined with zolpidem, these herbs may cause excessive drowsiness. Avoid sedative herbs such as chamomile (*Matricaria recutita*), catnip (*Nepeta cataria*), kava kava (*Piper methysticum*), passionflower (*Passiflora incarnata*), and valerian (*Valeriana officinalis*). St. John's wort (*Hypericum perforatum*). The combination of zolpidem and selective serotonin reuptake inhibitor (SSRI) drugs such as fluoxetine (see page 77) has been reported to cause hallucinations in some people. Because St. John's wort is thought to work in a way similar to SSRI drugs, it should not be used when taking zolpidem.
Bear in Mind:	Because of the interaction between zolpidem and selective serotonin reuptake inhibitor (SSRI) drugs (see above) experts advise against taking the natural sedatives 5-HTP, L-tryptophan, and SAMe when taking zolpidem because these supplements affect your serotonin levels. Zolpidem causes drowsiness. Alcohol makes this effect stronger. Don't use alcohol if taking this drug.